# A Guide to Active Working in the Modern Office

# A Guide to Active Working in the Modern Office

## Homo Sedens in the 21st Century

Robert Bridger

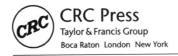

**CRC Press**
Taylor & Francis Group
Boca Raton  London  New York

CRC Press is an imprint of the
Taylor & Francis Group, an **informa** business

# *Dedication*

---

*A book for anyone wanting to be more active in the office.*

# Contents

# Preface

Is sitting really the new smoking as some have suggested and do we really need to sit less at work to be healthy? If we do, is standing any better? In this guide, I have reviewed research on standing and sitting going back almost 100 years to find some answers to these questions.

What is certain is that the physical demands of much of daily life nowadays bear no resemblance to those of our ancestors and are incompatible with what our bodies are designed to do. We have seen a steady rise in the prevalence of obesity in the general population and in health complaints such as Type II diabetes over the last 50 years. Coupled with an overabundance of cheap foods, dense in calories, the physical condition of the populations of many developed and developing countries has steadily deteriorated.

The human body is designed to survive famine and we crave sweet foods because they spare fat stores that are essential when food is scarce. In the past, the work of two people was needed to produce enough food for three and physical work varied with the seasons.

Office work is a new development in human history, but has been overtaken by technological and demographic changes.

Evidence is emerging that many of the adverse health effects of a sedentary lifestyle can be mitigated if offices and office work are designed to allow people to sit and stand naturally, the way they do in their free time (when not watching TV or playing computer games, of course!). Sit-stand desks and other new products can also play a role if people are prepared to use them.

To date, the scientific evidence that active workplace initiatives do reduce the time people spend sitting at work, is weak. However, that is not the same as saying that there is no evidence at all and that nothing can be done to make office work healthier. The weakness of the evidence is, in part, due to the difficulty of carrying out high-quality studies in real workplaces over long periods of time. There is plenty of experimental evidence to suggest that active workplace initiatives and better designs of furniture are *efficacious* (that is, beneficial in principle) but the evidence that they are *effective* (beneficial in practice and in the long term) is weaker.

In this guide, I have reviewed the scientific knowledge and evidence that there is and I have used it to provide the best information that I can at the time of writing. Each chapter ends with some key points and evidence-based guidance based on the material in the chapter.

I hope that this book will help you make informed decisions about whether and how to be more active at work.

# Author Biography

**Dr. Robert Bridger** is President of the Chartered Institute of Ergonomics and Human Factors and is an independent writer and consultant.

He has over 35 years of experience as a researcher and consultant in workplace and facilities design, safety and in education in ergonomics and human factors.

He is sole author of the textbook, *Introduction to Human Factors and Ergonomics*, now in its fourth edition and also published by CRC Press.

For more information about Dr. Bridger, visit www.rsbridger.com

# Acknowledgments

The author would like to thank the following for assistance with artwork and information:

Osmond Group Ltd. (www.ergonomics.co.uk)
Ergotron (www.ergotron.com)
noonee AG, Switzerland (www.venturekick.ch/noonee)
CoreChair Inc. (www.corechair.com)
Classroom seating solutions (www.footfidget.com)
Back in Action – The Back Shop, London, United Kingdom (www.backinaction.co.uk/)
TNO, dep. Healthy Living, the Netherlands (www.tno.nl/en/focus-areas/healthy-living/)
K2 Space, London, (hello@k2-space.co.uk)
StressNoMore.co.uk
Office Reality Ltd. (www.officereality.co.uk)
RAAAF architects, the Netherlands
British Broadcasting Corporation News Magazine
Pensinsula Technikon (Cape Town, South Africa)
Dr. A.C. Mandal

# 1 Posture and Movement in Everyday Life

"When Man assumed the upright position, he immediately made an enemy of gravity and has been fighting this relentless foe ever since."

**J.A. Jones (1933) quoted in Hellebrandt and Franseen (1943)**

One of the simplest ways to begin a book about being more active in the office is to start with the human body – what it is designed to do and how it works, with the emphasis on posture and movement.

Human beings are the last in a line of primates known as "hominins," which includes extinct human species such as Neanderthals and distant ancestors such as "Australopithicus." All were different from modern chimpanzees and gorillas in that the hominins were all well adapted to walking on two legs. Bipedalism is nothing new. One of the key differences between modern humans and other living primates is the ability to walk with the upper body in an upright position while taking long strides (Figure 1.1). The ability to do this is due, in part, to the shape of the human spine. In humans, the spine is "S"-shaped and there is a concave curve at the base of the spine (known as the "lumbar lordosis"). Five lumbar vertebrae curve inwards at the base of the spine, bending backwards to raise the upper body into an upright position over the pelvis and hip joints (Figure 1.2). The result is that the upper body is almost perfectly balanced over the bones and joints below.

Standing upright in this way is energy efficient – the energy expenditure of standing still isn't very much greater than when sitting in a chair or lying down. Why then, has it been proposed that "sitting is the new smoking" and that we should spend more time standing at work?

Standing to work at your computer instead of sitting all day has benefits, but "burning calories" isn't one of them.

We will explore this question in the following chapters. In this chapter, we will look at posture and movement in everyday life (when we can choose whether to stand, sit, walk or move) and how naturalistic postures differ from the postures normally adopted when we work in the office.

Humans are able to walk with a "striding gait" – we can take long strides because the hip joint of the trailing leg continues to extend as the other leg swings forwards.

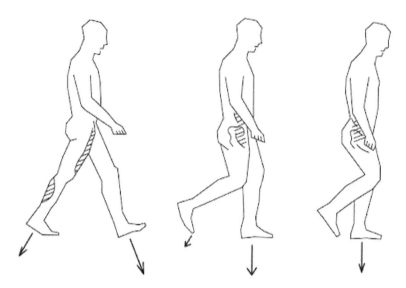

**FIGURE 1.1**  Humans are built to walk on two legs (bipedalism) taking long strides in an upright stance. The "S"-shaped spine in the lumbar region supports the weight of the upper body which is transmitted directly to the pelvis, hips, and knees. Walking is energy efficient even though we spend more than half of the time standing on one leg when we walk.

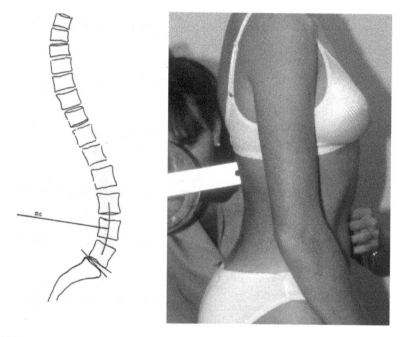

**FIGURE 1.2**  The spine seen from the side. In the upright position, the third lumbar vertebra is directly below the center of gravity of the upper body. The back and abdominal muscles do little work to maintain the upright posture because the mass of the upper body is balanced on the lumbar spine.

In fact, when we walk, we are standing on one leg more than half the time. One of the main anatomical differences in this respect between modern humans and chimpanzees and gorillas is that human beings are perfectly designed to stand on one leg – albeit for short periods of time. In a later chapter we will look at this in more detail and answer the question why, if we spend so much time standing on one leg when walking that we don't fall to one side or sway from side to side to maintain balance? For the moment, suffice to say that we are well adapted to walk on two legs and do so by standing on one leg more than half the time.

Standing still is associated with a host of problems both in the short term and in the long term (leg swelling, varicose veins and arthritis in the hip joints, (Bridger, 2018)), and we will look at these problems in a later chapter and find out how to avoid them. Only people who have to stand still ever do so – guardsmen, sentries, people engaged in ceremonial work or when washing the dishes (Figure 1.3). There

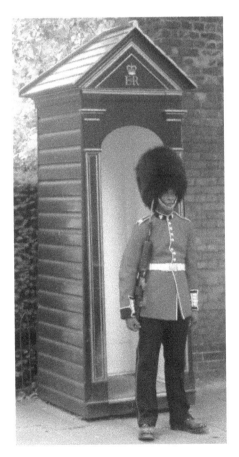

**FIGURE 1.3** Standing still is unnatural and is rarely seen in everyday life. Exceptions are jobs where people have to stand still for ceremonial reasons or as a transitional posture (e.g., when waiting for the traffic lights to indicate that it is safe to cross the road). (Source: Courtesy of Panhard: Queen's Guard, June 13, 2009, Wikimedia Commons, cropped.)

is a great deal of evidence that factory jobs, where people have to stand in the same place all day long are harmful and increase the risk of ill health in later life. Standing still, when it does occur in everyday life is a transitional posture that is momentarily adopted when finishing one activity and starting another – for example, when standing by the road waiting for the traffic lights to indicate that it is safe to cross.

## NATURAL STANDING

Standing upright is a constant challenge for three reasons – firstly the need to maintain balance on an unstable base with only two points of support for the body (the feet); secondly the need to avoid discomfort due to static loading of joints and muscles and thirdly the need to return blood from the lower limbs back to the heart against gravity.

Standing on two legs is the exception rather than the rule in the animal kingdom. Animals that do stand on two legs have anatomical adaptations to help them maintain balance. The long tail of the kangaroo counterbalances its upper body when it moves and acts as a third leg when it is stationary. Humans don't have tails, so they use external objects as a third base of support to stabilize the body (Figure 1.4).

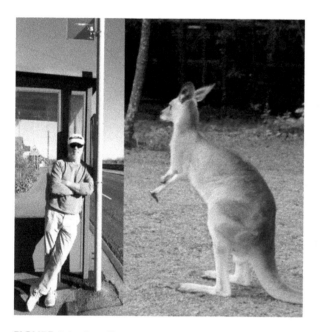
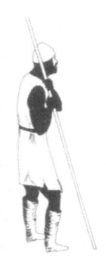

**FIGURE 1.4**    Standing on two legs is the exception rather than the rule in the animal kingdom. Kangaroos, although largely bipedal, use their tails as a "third leg" to achieve a tripedal standing posture that is much more stable. Humans lean against objects to increase stability and transfer some of the body weight to other parts of the body (the shoulder in this example). Standing still with the arms dangling by the sides is uncomfortable. Folding the arms and crossing the legs are postural strategies that we use to close these open chains and stabilize them with friction, enabling the muscles to relax. (Source: Kangaroo photo by Blacktator from Pexels.

In humans, the lumbar lordosis (the inward curve of the lower back in the lumbar region) supports the weight of the upper body in an energy efficient way. When people stand for a long time, fatigue, when it occurs, is not due to increased energy expenditure but compression of soft tissues and pooling of blood in the lower legs. Typically, people use postural strategies to stabilize themselves and avoid discomfort as in Figure 1.4.

## THINGS PEOPLE DO WHEN STANDING NATURALLY

1. Never stand still
2. Shift body weight on one leg
3. Lean backwards against anything
4. Lean sideways against a vertical surface
5. Rest hip against counters
6. Maximize contact with fixed objects
7. Use arms as props resting elbows on a surface
8. Place one foot on a raised surface
9. Use thoracic support (e.g., lean on a broom)
10. Hang on elbows
11. Rest upper body on a counter
12. Place hands on hips or in pockets
13. Sit on heels against a wall
14. Use a footrest
15. Sit down whenever possible
16. Extend footprint
17. Rest chin on hand
18. Rest knee on surface
19. Rest hands on knees
20. Fold arms, cross legs at the ankles (list taken from Bridger et al., 1994).

At work, the opportunity to use these strategies, to stand and move naturally, is diminished due to the demands of the work and the design of the furniture. This is one of the reasons, although not the only one, why sedentary work became so common in the late 19th and early 20th centuries. It wasn't practical to expect thousands of office workers to stand still all day doing clerical work.

Gravity won and the seated work position became the norm.

## AVOIDING DISCOMFORT

The heaviest load most of us will ever have to carry in our entire lives is our own body. In everyday life people use postural strategies to minimize the load, particularly the load on the joints, and also to minimize the effort required to move and carry out tasks.

We can think of posture, *as the way we carry ourselves*. So the postures we adopt everyday can have a very large effect on the effort we have to expend in performing daily activities. Posture also has a very large effect on the forces that act on the muscles and joints of the body, including those of the spine. Posture is all about body mechanics.

So, what is a "good posture"?

The short answer is that there is no "good" posture. All postures in daily life impose compressive and tensile stresses on tissues and interfere with the flow of blood to some tissues and not others. This explains why most people, when left to their own devices, make small postural adjustments all the time.

But some postures *are* better than others – the "better" postures enable us to carry ourselves efficiently, expending the minimum of effort as we do so, without unnecessary strain. In daily life, we are normally completely unaware of our posture and how the body automatically adapts to the demands we place on it.

## STANDING STILL (OR TRYING TO)

When we stand still with our feet together, the body is like an inverted pendulum. It is a tall structure with a narrow base of support. The center of gravity of the body lies at more than half its total height. Two sets of reflexes act to keep us upright. The antigravity reflexes are essential for upright posture. They contract to "brace" the joints against gravity. A second set of postural reflexes controls the positions of the various body parts in relation to each other (postural fixation of limbs, for example) and the posture of the whole body itself.

Some quadrupedal animals can "lock" their limbs to achieve stability at little energy cost (apparently, this is one reason why horses can sleep standing up).

In humans, stability is achieved dynamically. Viewed from the side, the anterior and posterior muscles of the body (those at the front and the back) act to keep the center of gravity (COG) of the body within the small base of support defined by the position of the feet. Foot position is a critical determinant of posture and plays an important role in standing workplace design. It has been found that people will adopt an asymmetrical standing attitude four times as often as a symmetrical stance. When standing naturally, the body weight is supported almost entirely on one leg while the other assists in maintaining balance (Smith, 1953).

Postural reflexes act so that, for example, forward flexion of the upper body in front of the feet is accompanied by posterior projection of the buttocks to maintain balance (Figure 1.5).

Try this simple demonstration to get a feel for "postural adaptation."

Stand in the middle of a room and look straight ahead. Place your hands on your hip joints (about the level of your trouser pockets, at the top of your legs), and lean forwards, keeping your back straight and *without moving your feet*. Hold this position for a few seconds, then straighten up and relax.

Now move to the side of the room and stand with your back to the wall and your heels against the wall. Repeat the bending movement you performed previously.

What happens? You can't bend forwards very far without becoming unstable and you have to either straighten up or take a step forwards to regain stability.

Figure 1.5 demonstrates the body mechanics involved. When we stand upright in a comfortable position, the weight of our body lies above our feet. This is no different from saying that the weight of the food on a laden dinner table lies within the

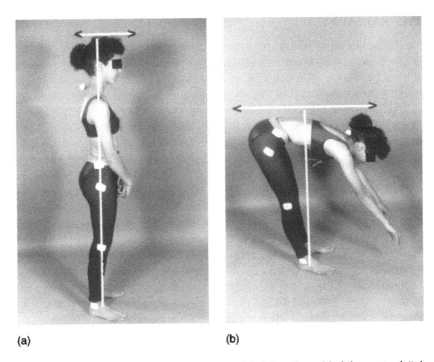

(a)                                                    (b)

**FIGURE 1.5**   When we lean forwards from the hip joint, the ankle joints extend ('plan-tarflex' to use anatomical terminology) to compensate and the buttocks and legs move in the opposite direction to the upper body to maintain balance. Compensatory movements like these take place all the time in everyday life and we are normally not aware of them. Only when badly designed workplaces or lack of space prevent normal postural compensation do we become aware that something is wrong.

base of support provided by the table legs. If you remove one of the table legs, the table will tilt and the food will fall onto the floor.

When you stood in the middle of the room and flexed forwards, the weight of your upper body started to move forwards towards the toe-end of your foot support base. You probably weren't aware of it at the time, but your lower body automatically compensated for this weight shift. Your ankles extended and your hip joints, legs and buttocks moved in the opposite direction. The reason it did this was to keep the center of gravity of the whole body above the feet evenly balanced over the base.

What you have just observed is an example of *postural adaptation*. Most postural adaptation in daily life takes place automatically and we are not aware of it. It was only when you stood against the wall and tried to flex forwards that you noticed the difference – the wall blocked the postural adaptation and the only way to flex forwards without falling forwards is to move one foot forwards and/or bend the knees.

*When standing at work, then, we need to ensure that there is plenty of space around the feet for standing workers so that they can change posture and maintain good balance.*

## POSTURAL SWAY

In healthy people under less drastic circumstances, relaxed standing is accompanied by postural sway. We are not normally aware of postural sway, but sway is exaggerated when people are intoxicated or are about to faint. Even when we think we are standing still, we are swaying slightly and balance is maintained by the action of muscle reflexes and supplemented by vision.

Several factors influence postural stability and sway in healthy people. Age has been found to be related to sway in some studies but not in others. Women tend to have better balance than men, possibly because they have a lower center of gravity. Vision is an important stabilizing factor that helps us to stand still (we are more likely to lose balance in poor lighting) whereas severe hearing loss has been shown to correlate with increased sway. Standing on one leg while blindfolded is very difficult for most people (and impossible for most people over 55 years of age). Standing on one leg without a blindfold is more difficult than standing with the feet together with a blindfold. These results are not surprising in view of the reduction in the size of the base of support, increased muscle coordination (recruitment of the hip abductors, the muscles at the side of the hip joint to maintain the center of gravity of the body over a single foot) and loss of visual feedback brought about by this test.

Postural sway is reduced when we look at a fixed target that is directly ahead – such as a computer screen – and the lack of movement quickly leads to fatigue.

## THE "ANTIGRAVITY" MUSCLES AND POSTURAL SWAY

Unlike quadrupedal animals, which support themselves on four legs, humans stand on two – the base of support for the body as described by the position of the feet is much smaller in humans than in quadrupeds. Standing is inherently unstable and is maintained by a group of muscles known as the "antigravity muscles." The center of gravity of the body as a whole is just above the hip joint. In relaxed standing, the upper body is supported by the skeleton and stabilized by the action of the antigravity muscles.

An "ankle strategy" is used to counter small perturbations of the COG and a "hip strategy" to counter large perturbations or when the support surface is narrow (when working in a confined space or on a narrow plank for example). For posterior displacements (leaning backwards), the muscles on the front of the lower leg and thigh contract (tibialis anterior and quadriceps femoris) in the ankle strategy, and the paraspinal and hamstring muscles in the hip strategy. So, standing in any kind of posture that is unbalanced will place additional load on some or all of the antigravity muscles and lead to discomfort.

One of the main postural strategies for dealing with loss of balance when the hip and ankle strategies fail, is to correct the loss of balance by moving the feet to extend the base of support for the body. If the foot space is restricted due to the design of the workspace or clutter on the floor, losses of balance are more likely.

## DEMONSTRATION OF THE ANTIGRAVITY MUSCLES IN ACTION

For a practical demonstration of postural sway, try standing on one leg for 20 seconds, then close your eyes (not recommended for people over 55 years of age).

In relaxed standing, the skeleton can be likened to the poles of a tent, the muscles to the guy ropes and the skin to the canvas (Figure 1.6). The tension in the muscles, like the tension in the guy ropes of a tent should be in balance.

The main challenge in remaining upright in the symmetrical (feet together) position is maintaining the high body center of gravity over a small support base.

Try this simple demonstration. Stand in a relaxed posture. Place one hand over the muscles in your lower back and look straight ahead. Place the other hand over your abdomen. In a relaxed standing position, you should feel that you are carrying your body weight on your heels and the muscles in your lower back and stomach should feel relaxed.

The back muscles should not be tense. Now, lean forward from the ankle joints – feel the weight of your body move towards your toes. The lower back muscles will tense as the weight of the upper body moves away from them. Now lean back as the weight moves over your heels. The back muscles relax and the abdominal muscles start to contract.

If you get backache when working at a standing desk, it might be due to muscle fatigue caused by leaning forwards to reach work objects. Check that your keyboard

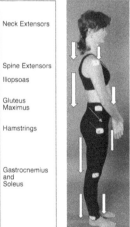
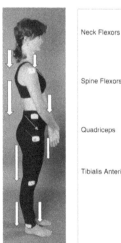
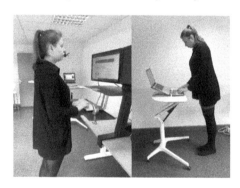

**FIGURE 1.6** If the skeleton is like the poles of a tent, the antigravity muscles are akin to the guy ropes. When standing to work at a computer, little muscle activity is needed if the screen and keyboard are at the correct height and distance from the body. If they are too low, the user has to lean forwards, and the antigravity muscles at the back have to contract to maintain the position. To avoid discomfort when working at a standing desk, change the layout of the desk to suit the posture – don't change the posture to suit the layout. The screen should be no higher than your eyes and no lower than 30 degrees below the line of sight. The keyboard should be the same height as your elbows.

is no more than about 40cm in front of your body and directly in front of you (this is called the "zone of convenient reach") and that you can work with your upper arms at your sides and relaxed.

Leaning forward places a constant static load on the back muscles, which causes backache when the muscles become fatigued. *If you stand too far away from your keyboard when working at a standing desk, you may find it difficult to maintain a relaxed standing posture, tension in the back muscles will result and lead to backache. Better to push the keyboard back from the desk, making sure the screen is at a comfortable viewing distance, and stand close to the desk so that you can rest your elbows on the desktop.*

## SITTING AROUND THE WORLD

According to Hewes (1957) humans are capable of adopting over 1000 comfortable working and resting postures but, given the freedom to do so, only adopt any particular posture for short periods of time. In most cultures, however, only a subset of postures is practiced due to tradition, climate and terrain, clothing design and the methods of work. The most widely researched posture is undoubtedly standing followed by the Western "90-degree" sitting posture, as well as its reclining variants and the furniture used to support it.

Standing is universal but the same cannot be said for sitting in chairs. This has its origin in Ancient Greece and Egypt, where only those with high social status sat on chairs. The rest of the population appears to have sat on the floor or on low stools. A common posture, worldwide, is the deep squat shown in Figure 1.7.

Squatting is the habitual resting position of the chimpanzee and is readily adopted by young children of any culture. In Western societies, children usually lose the ability to squat soon after starting school because they spend a large part of the day sitting on chairs when they start school (Milne and Mireau, 1979). Part of the reason for the loss of the ability to squat is a reduction on the distensibility (flexibility) of the hamstring and other muscles which become shortened when

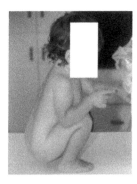 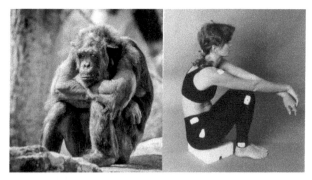

**FIGURE 1.7**  Squatting is the habitual resting posture of the chimpanzee and is readily adopted by young children. The ability to squat comfortably appears to be lost when children attend schools and sit on chairs. In the Western world, most adults have to compensate for the loss of flexibility when they attempt to squat.

squatting is replaced by sitting. Adults not accustomed to squatting find it difficult for the same reasons. Many adults in Western societies can't flex their ankles sufficiently to bring the center of gravity of the body over the feet and therefore tend to fall backwards when attempting to squat. On those occasions where squatting is achieved, it is by squatting "on the toes" to compensate for the reduced flexibility in the calf muscles, by sitting on something or with the back supported by leaning against a wall.

Squatting was regarded as vulgar by the Ancient Greeks, which may explain why it is not practiced in countries influenced by their culture and traditions. However, millions of people in many parts of Asia, Africa, Latin America and Oceania customarily work and rest in this position – the center of gravity of the body is low, directly above the feet and is therefore stable.

Cross-legged sitting is common in North Africa, the Middle East, India, South East Asia and Indonesia and also Korea, Japan and Polynesia. It is depicted in ancient Mayan sculptures and in the pottery of many tribes of North and South America. Convention, clothing and cold, damp floors restrict its use in Western culture (although it is a common posture in schoolchildren and was the working posture of English tailors until relatively recently) but most people are able to sit in this way. The hips are flexed, abducted and laterally rotated with the knees resting on the foot of the opposite leg. The two-joint muscles of the hip are relaxed as is iliopsoas (a muscle connecting the thigh bone to the pelvis and lumbar spine) and body weight is born by the ischia (seat bones) and not the coccyx. In India there are many variations of this basic position. According to Sen (1984) some of the benefits of sitting cross-legged on the floor while working are as follows:

1. Improved blood flow from the legs ("venous return")
2. A more desirable resting position for the hip joints
3. Avoidance of the need to lift objects onto raised surfaces
4. More postural options (given an appropriate floor surface).

"Long sitting" (sitting on the floor with a 90-degree angle between the trunk and the thighs with the knees extended) is a common working and resting posture among women in Africa, Melanesia, South East Asia and Indian North West America.

Sitting on the heels with the knees resting on the floor is a formal sitting posture for both men and women in Japan. It is the position for praying in the Islamic world. In Africa, Mexico and parts of South East Asia it is mainly used by women. It appears to have been a working posture used to grind corn in ancient times where women would use a stone to grind the corn against a larger stone slab on the floor. Ancient Egyptian scribes sometimes adopted this posture when writing. Most adults in Western culture can attain this posture even without practice, except those with overdeveloped or tight quadriceps muscles or knee injuries. Of the nine sitting and standing postures investigated by Bridger et al. (1992a) this was the posture of least constraint of the hip joint with the lumbar spine and pelvis in the middle of their ranges.

Sitting on the floor is generally unacceptable in Western society and it is interesting to observe that a very similar posture was implemented in a more acceptable form – as a piece of furniture which lifts the user off the floor to desk height (Figure 1.8).

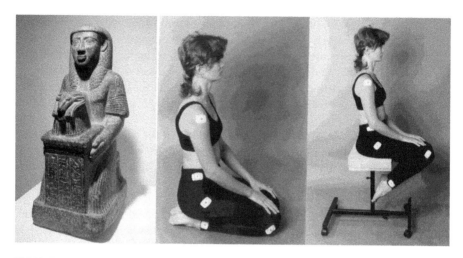

**FIGURE 1.8** Kneeling statue of Yupa, Pharoah Ramesses II's scribe, Egypt, New Kingdom, 19th dynasty c. 1279–1213 BC, black granite (Exhibit in the Krannert Art Museum, University of Illinois at Urbana-Champaign, Illinois, USA.). A kneeling chair for writing at a desk.

## POSTURE AND BACK PAIN

There is *some* truth in the generalization that there are four types of people in the world (see Figure 1.9 for further explanation):

1. Those who rarely get back pain (the lucky few).
2. People who get back pain when bending or leaning forwards (often due to degenerated lumbar intervertebral discs that generate pain symptoms, partly as a result of genetic predisposition to disc degeneration (Kalichman and Hunter, 2008)).
3. Those with problems in the joints at the rear of the spine (facet joints at C in Figure 1.9). People with disc problems often get back pain when leaning forwards over a desk, sitting for long periods or during activities such as gardening. People with facet joint problems often get back pain when standing or during activities that accentuate the lumbar curve.
4. Those unfortunate few with chronic pain syndromes where the pain has little to do with posture and movement in everyday life except to limit what the sufferers are able to do.

## DEGENERATION OF THE SPINE AND EVERYDAY LIFE

Several investigations of the incidence of spinal pathology have been carried out in different societies in different parts of the world. Fahrni and Trueman (1965) compared the incidence of degenerative changes in the spine in North Americans and Europeans and a jungle-dwelling tribe in India. In all groups, degeneration of the spine in the lumbar region increased with age, but the trends were steeper for the

anterior elements                                                 posterior elements

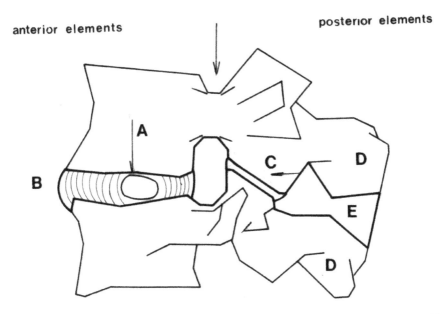

**FIGURE 1.9** Side view of lumbar vertebrae (A) and intervertebral disc (B). People with symptomatic discs often find postures that flex the spine, such as slumped sitting postures, cause pain. People with degeneration of the facet joints (C) may find standing or kneeling painful. There is no "one size fits all" solution to the problem of back pain in the workplace.

Western groups than the Indian tribe. The incidence of intervertebral disc degeneration was much less among the Indians and was hardly age-related at all. This may have something to do with the more varied postures adopted at different times of the day in pre-industrial societies.

Fahrni and Trueman noted that the spines of horses, cows, dogs, camels and giraffes degenerate at levels where the mechanical strain is greatest – the upper back and neck (cervico-thoracic region) of camels and giraffes, the lower thoracic level in the basset hound and dachshund dog and the apex of the lumbar spine in humans.

Studies of the fossilized remains of the giant dinosaur diplodocus suggest that degeneration of its spine occurred in the tail which it used as a prop when standing on its hind legs (Blumberg and Sokoloff, 1961).

Suffice to say that spinal problems tend to be more common in those parts of the spine that are exposed to the highest mechanical loads in everyday life. In humans, these are the lumbar spine (pain in the low back, sometimes referred to as "lumbago") and the cervical spine (pain in the back of the neck). In flexed sitting postures (sitting "hunched" over the desk, as in Figure 1.10) the lumbar discs are stressed and the neck muscles have to maintain the head with the cervical spine in a flexed position and under load. When standing, the posterior elements in Figure 1.9 (the facet joints) take more of the load (Adams et al., 2002).

In everyday life and given the freedom to do so, people avoid postures that place a high load on the spine and change posture frequently to redistribute the load, as we shall see in the next section.

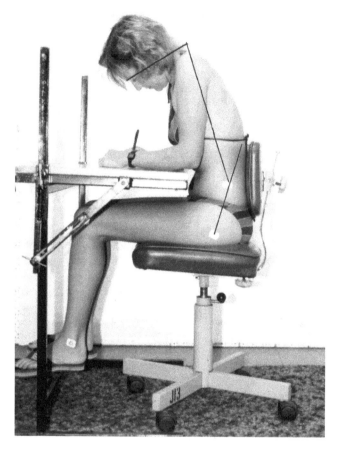

**FIGURE 1.10**  Slumped sitting posture – a common cause of backache in people with symptomatic lumbar discs and neckache due to fatigue in the muscles of the neck. Standing to work for short periods may delay or prevent the onset of discomfort.

When standing to work with computers in the office, screens placed too high can increase the load on the cervical spine and accentuate the lumbar curve which increases the load in the facet joints and may cause pain (Figure 1.11).

## POSTURAL BEHAVIOR IN EVERYDAY LIFE

The human body can be thought of as an open chain of linked segments consisting of bones, joints and the muscles crossing the joints (Dempster, 1955). In order to move and to carry out useful functional movements, each joint of the body has a freedom for motion in one or more directions. A complex linkage, such as that between the shoulder, arm and hand has many degrees of freedom of movement, and power transmission is impossible without stabilization of joints by muscle action. For example, try threading a needle with your hands held out in front of your body, with arms extended. The main effort is maintaining the posture, not threading the

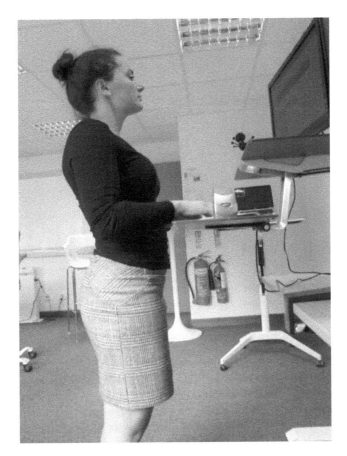

**FIGURE 1.11**  Working at a standing desk with the screen too high can cause uncomfort-able postural deviations – note the exaggerated lumbar curve (excessive lordosis) and the strained neck posture (chin held high to look at the screen).

needle. When turning a door handle, for example, the force is exerted by the hand by turning the wrist. But this is only possible if the elbow and shoulder joints are stabilized by the muscles around them – otherwise the handle would remain still and the arm would move instead.

## CLOSING THE CHAIN – WHY DO WE FOLD OUR ARMS AND CROSS OUR LEGS?

Why do people habitually fold their arms or cross their legs? The main reason seems to be to close the chain and stabilize the limbs by friction, which enables the mus-cles to relax. In the absence of this kind of stabilization, low level muscle activity of which we are seldom aware is required. So, postural strategies such as folding the arms and crossing the legs enable the muscles surrounding the joints to relax (Figure 1.12). Snijders et al. (1995) found that the abdominal muscles were more

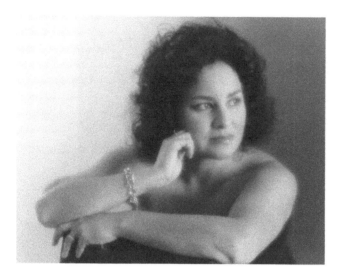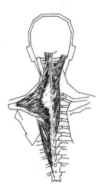

**FIGURE 1.12**    The neck extensor muscles are antigravity muscles that maintain the head in an upright position. When relaxing, we use the arms as props to support the upper body and the neck by cupping the chin in the hand. This is a common postural strategy seen in everyday life – it enables the extensor muscles of the neck and upper back to relax.

relaxed when seated people crossed their legs, possibly because crossing the legs stabilizes the pelvis from below so the upper body rests on a more stable base.

We interact with objects around us for the same reason – for example, using our upper arms as props to support the weight of the upper body when sitting at a table. These postural strategies are perceived as restful and we unconsciously adopt them for short periods whenever we are able to do so (Figure 1.12).

## INDUSTRIAL SITTING AND STANDING

One of the reasons why deskbound office workers get aches and pains is the lack of postural change. When fully engaged with work at a computer or laptop, there may be few options to change posture. Despite the best intentions of furniture designers and facilities managers, static postures are common with increased risk of health complaints (Figure 1.13).

The prime function of a chair is to support the weight of the body by spreading the load over the seat and backrest. A second function is to stabilize the limbs. The comfort of a seat or any other piece of furniture, therefore, depends on the extent to which it permits muscular relaxation while stabilizing the limbs.

As we shall see in Chapter 4, these requirements for comfortable working throughout the day, *also reduce energy expenditure.*

*Much of the focus on office furniture design in the last 40 years has been on providing comfortable workspaces for sedentary computer users. It now seems that success in doing so has contributed a different set of problems associated with physical inactivity*

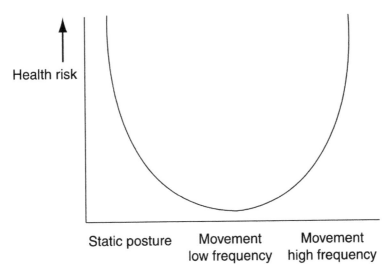

**FIGURE 1.13**  Health risk at work depends on avoiding long periods of inactivity such as standing still or static exertions such as bending. A moderate amount of postural variety lowers the risk. (Source: Bridger (2018), with permission.)

As we shall see in the chapters that follow, there is a trade-off between providing comfortable working conditions on the one hand, while maintaining a suitable level of physical activity on the other. Standing may have advantages over sitting in the modern office but a better way to think about it is that *both can bring their own problems*. These problems can be tackled by following the guidance in the rest of this book.

## KEY POINTS

1. We are capable of over 1000 comfortable work and restful postures but typically only adopt any particular posture for a short period of time.
2. The heaviest load most of us will ever carry is our own body and in daily life we constantly seek ways of reducing the load.
3. The spines of animals tend to fail in the regions that are exposed to the highest loads. In humans, these are the lumbar and cervical regions.
4. We adopt postural strategies to reduce low level muscle activity needed to maintain posture. These are expressed as postural behaviors such as folding the arms, crossing the legs and leaning against objects.
5. There is no such thing as a "correct" posture but some postures are better than others. Sitting or standing still for long periods are not examples of the better postures.
6. Don't use the space underneath standing desks for storage – it steals foot space and limits the number of postures people can adopt when standing.

7. Place work objects (keyboards, the mouse etc.) no more than 40cm away from the body when standing to work at a computer.

8. Both standing and sitting can bring their own problems, particularly if the workspace is set up incorrectly (Figures 1.10 and 1.11). Incorrect workspace design can affect back sufferers in different ways, depending on the source of the symptoms.

9. Change posture throughout the day to avoid backache. The ability to change from sitting to standing favors the use of "sit-stand" workstations.

# 2 Why Do We Sit in the Office?

## Seating as a Solution

*The chief idea in our system, as in his, is, that the* authority for doing all kinds *of work should proceed from one central office to the various departments, and that there proper records should be kept of the work and reports made daily to the central office, so that the superintending department should be kept thoroughly informed as to what is taking place throughout the works, and at the same time no work could be done in the works without proper authority.*

**F.W. Taylor (1886), "Comment to 'The Shop-Order System of Accounts,' " by Henry Metcalfe in *Transactions of the American Society of Mechanical Engineers*, Vol 7 (1885–1886), p. 475; partly cited in Wrege and Greenwood (1991), p. 204**

Prior to the Industrial Revolution, most of the population of Europe were illiterate and were engaged in manual work. According to some authorities, in Northern Europe, it took the work of two people to produce enough to feed three. Sedentary work was the exception rather than the rule and the forerunners of today's offices were the Monastic Scriptoria of medieval times. Figure 2.1 shows a 9th-century ivory relief depicting Pope Gregory the Great and his scribes.

Has sedentary work always been a problem? Nicolas Andry de Bois-Regard (1658–1742) one of the founding fathers of occupational medicine and orthopedics, thought sitting upright to be a "good posture" whereas sitting hunched forwards over a desk (with the spine flexed) was a "bad posture" with the back "crooked and round" and "ungraceful."

The ivory relief depicts the Pope at work hunched over his desk in what appears to be a very uncomfortable posture. It is likely that the artist depicted the task in this way in order to emphasize the piety and dedication of St Gregory in enduring physical discomfort in order to complete his task. Other depictions of medieval scribes show chairs and desks with similar design features, but different proportions. The sloping desk is normally much higher as is the chair – more akin to a draughtsman's worktable in modern times and, very likely, more historically accurate.

Nevertheless, one of the 1000-year-old lessons to be learned from this ivory relief is that when the visual and manual requirements of a task are not well met by the

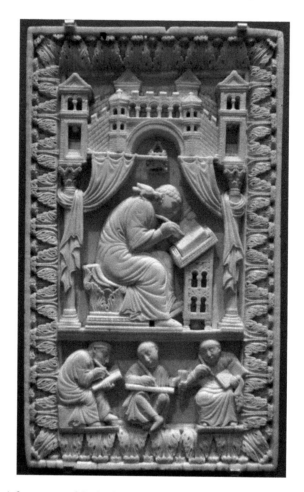

**FIGURE 2.1**   A forerunner of the 20th-century office? Saint Gregory the Great with scribes. Note the hunched and cramped posture, flexed spine, extended neck with the chin protruding, suggesting the work is visually demanding or the lighting poor. The left hand steadies the book and the right hand works on the manuscript. The artist may have taken license here to depict an unhealthy static posture to underline the piety of the Saint. Late 9th-century ivory relief from the cover of a sacramentary, now in the Kunsthistorisches Museum in Vienna.

design of the furniture, postural and visual problems occur which can lead to the development of long-term health complaints. The Pope has to adapt his posture to suit the workspace – the modern view, of course, is that workspaces should be adaptable to meet the needs of users.

In the 17th and 18th centuries, office work was conducted to support the activities of merchants and government officials. Early offices were modeled on drawing rooms of the houses of wealthy or the work was conducted in coffee houses (Figure 2.2).

Standing desks, partly descended from the pulpits of medieval churches, were quite common in early factories and it was not unusual for managers and supervisors to work standing at a desk while clerks and assistants worked seated.

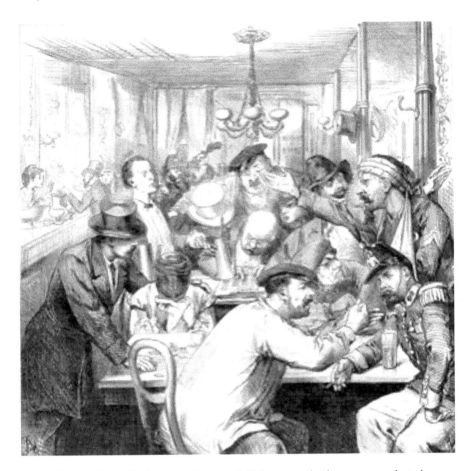

**FIGURE 2.2** The coffee house – where much 18th-century business was conducted.

In the Victorian era, there was a great deal of interest in furniture design – particularly school furniture, as state-sponsored compulsory schooling was introduced in many countries. Millions of children began to spend a large proportion of their childhood sitting at school desks. Medical experts and designers produced many new designs of school furniture with admirable design features: lumbar supports, footrests and sloping work surfaces – all to promote what was believed to be a healthy posture in schoolchildren.

Figure 2.3 shows an early example of a "sit-stand" school desk for children designed in 1879. There is nothing new about the idea that people should be able to carry out the same desk-based tasks when sitting or standing. One of the more admirable features of the sit-stand desk in the figure is that it supports three different postures – sitting, standing and an intermediate "semi-standing" posture – half way between sitting and standing. This posture is rarely seen in offices but is common in factories where workstations are designed to allow standing and "semi-standing" (Figure 2.4). Semi-standing is also popular with people who engage in field sports and take "shooting sticks" with them (walking sticks with a handle that folds into a seat).

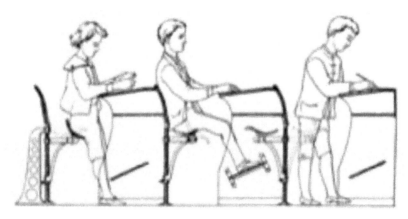

**FIGURE 2.3** Sit-stand school desk (Schindler 1890) – note also the sloping worktop for reading and writing to encourage upright standing and sitting postures. Schindler's school desk features many of the requirements for a sit-stand workstation. (Source: Burgerstein and Netolitzky, 1985.)

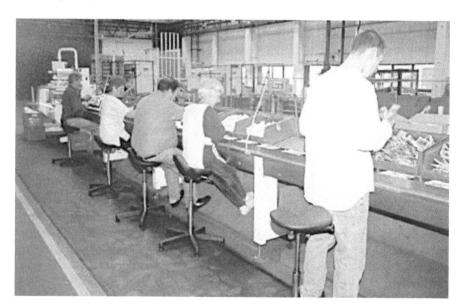

**FIGURE 2.4**    Standing and semi-standing in a modern factory.

So, with so many different ideas for the design of seated workspaces and standing desks already well-established, why did sedentary office work become the norm?

## WHY DID SEDENTARY WORK BECOME THE NORM?

With the development of railways and the expansion of international commerce and trade, with vastly increased markets and over much greater distances, the amount of paperwork needed to conduct business grew rapidly. New building techniques such as steel frame construction led to the forerunners of modern office buildings, making possible unobstructed, cathedral-like open spaces. There were immediate advantages for lighting and ventilation. Early air conditioning systems needed large spaces to function effectively therefore a large, centralized system of work was more practical. No longer did the head office of a company resemble the town house of a wealthy aristocrat. By the turn of the 20th century, new buildings emerged whose sole purpose was to process large volumes of paperwork in the most efficient way possible (Figure 2.5). It is important to emphasize that these early 20th-century office designs were geared to meet the requirement to process and move large volumes of paper through different departments. The office was a "paperwork" factory, hence the need for large spaces, unobstructed by walls and partitions. Some offices even had conveyor belts to move documents from one stage of processing to another (Sundstrom, 1986).

The Larkin Administration Building was designed in 1904 by the architect Frank Lloyd Wright for the Larkin Soap Company, which ran a mail order business from its factory. The five-story building was very advanced for its time with air conditioning, mechanical ventilation, stained glass windows and built-in office furniture made of metal. It was the first air-conditioned building in the United States. Another innovation was the central atrium with a glass skylight allowing clerical workers,

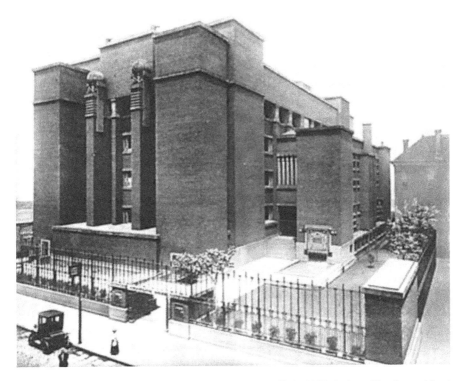

**FIGURE 2.5** The Larkin Administration Building built in 1908 designed by the architect Frank Lloyd Wright. A factory for processing paperwork and possibly one of the earliest truly modern offices.

with no view from a window, some natural daylight and supplementing the artificial light from the aisles. Managers worked around the perimeter of the Atrium in private offices with glass partitions and had a view from a window. A staff canteen was situated on the 5th floor (Figure 2.6).

Together with the new building techniques came a new style of management. At the time, the forerunners of modern Industrial Engineering were the disciplines

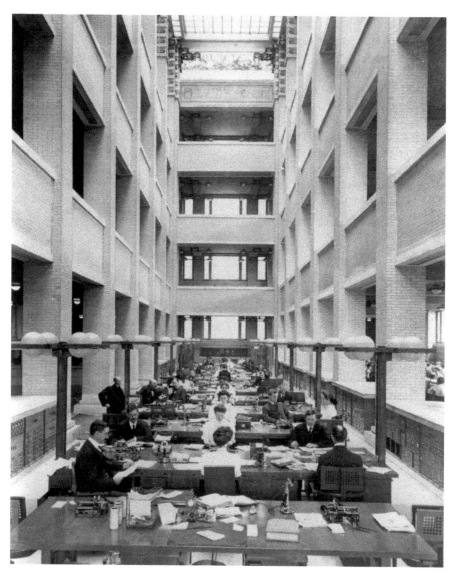

**FIGURE 2.6** Larkin Administration Building. Interior of the Larkin Administration Building, central court looking south showing employees at work. (Source: Courtesy of the collection of The Buffalo History Museum. Larkin Company photograph collection, Picture .L37, # 1–35.)

of "Scientific Management" and "Work Study." The newly emerging paperwork factories at the turn of the 20th century were organized around management principles popularized by these disciplines, which emphasized the division of labor and the standardization of tasks. F.W. Taylor in his 1911 book promoted the ideas of "Scientific Management" – in particular, that there was "one best way" of performing a task (Taylor, 1911). Once this method had been identified and defined, work station designs and layout, supervision, bonus schemes and the work environment would all be designed to enable the task to be conducted as efficiently as possible by a "top-down" system of management built around a rigid hierarchy.

One of the key principles of Scientific Management was a strong focus on standardization – of methods, of completion times for tasks and of equipment including chairs and desks, which were mass-produced. Workers were "tied to their desks" and closely supervised while they carried out repetitive, time-based tasks.

The office was a paperwork factory (Figures 2.7) and the chair made its debut as a piece of industrial furniture.

The Larkin Building is an excellent example of one of these "early office factories." It was purpose built to provide:

- A communal work experience
- Convenient means of supervision (because the job content required strict adherence to rules and procedures)
- A work environment to promote efficiency (at the time, mechanical ventilation systems and air conditioning only worked in large spaces)
- Unobstructed work flow.

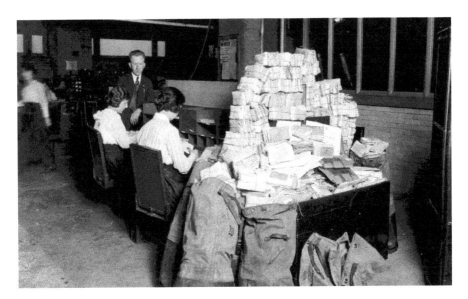

**FIGURE 2.7** The office as a paperwork factory. Mail room Larkin Company Administration Building, June 1920. (Source: Courtesy of the collection of The Buffalo History Museum. Larkin Company photograph collection, Picture .L37, #2–29.)

Another modern feature of the building which was subsequently adopted in many other buildings was the advantage of it being "one great loft" subdivided by light, interchangeable panels. Owners could maximize occupancy and the occupants could subdivide the space to suit themselves. However, there were also disadvantages due to the lack of flexibility to suit the requirements of individuals and workgroups.

## NEW JOBS FOR THE NEW OFFICES

Typewriters were developed to mechanize and standardize writing. The first commercially successful typewriter appeared in the USA in 1878. Typewriters were widely adopted and brought rapid improvements in the speed of production and the quality of the documents produced (Figure 2.8).

This change in the way documents were produced led to the creation of new jobs – typists and stenographers. Many women were attracted to these roles for a variety of reasons, not least because the working conditions in offices such as the Larkin Building were usually far superior to those in factories and the work was less physically demanding. Typing was also considered to be a "respectable" occupation for women. It is characteristic of the time that typists were considered to be skilled machine operators and it was soon recognized that formal training

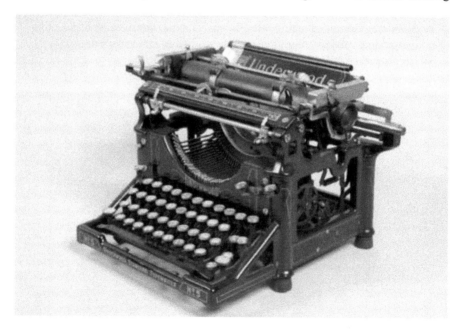

**FIGURE 2.8** The Underwood No. 5 typewriter was a fixture in businesses in the early 20th century. Designed in 1901 by Frank Wagner, typists soon preferred this speedy and reliable machine. In 1900 the company published an ad boasting that the U.S. Navy purchased 250 of them. (Source: Courtesy of The Children's Museum of Indianapolis, IMCPL Digital Collections (The Children&#039;s Museum of Indianapolis [CC BY-SA 3.0 (https://creative-commons.org/licenses/by-sa/3.0]).)

was needed to ensure that they used the "correct" method of typing to achieve a set production standard most efficiently. Skilled typists could produce up to 130 words per minute.

It was also recognized that specialized furniture would need to be provided to suit the needs of the mainly female workforce of typists (Figure 2.9). Desks for typewriters were typically lower than standard desks used for reading and writing because the keys on the keyboard were 10cm or more above the desktop. Typists chairs were designed with lumbar supports to support an upright sitting posture, with space for the buttocks to protrude at the rear; seats had limited depth from front to back to ensure that the weight of the upper body was supported by the "seat bones" (ischial tuberosities) and not by the soft tissues under the thighs. Typists were trained how to sit at their machines and how to adjust their furniture to achieve the "correct" working posture. In fact, much of the advice given to typists in those days would be considered to be good ergonomics even today. No doubt it benefited the health and wellbeing of the typists as well as their productivity.

A U.S. Navy Instructional Film of 1944 (Basic Typing, Part 1: Bureau of Aeronautics, Division of Personnel Supervision and Management, 1944) explained to trainee typists the key workstation requirements for a comfortable and efficient way of working.

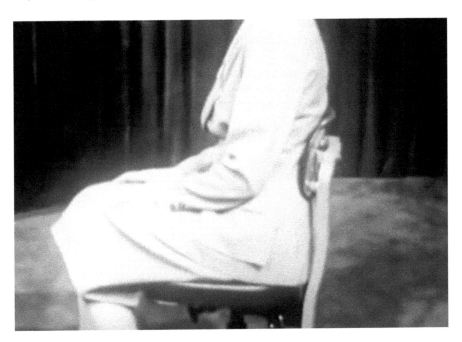

**FIGURE 2.9** Typist's chair, 1940s. Copy typing was ubiquitous until the 1980s. Copy typists were trained to type without reading the text. The task was simply to convert handwritten text into type. They were trained to adjust and sit on furniture designed for the purpose (from U.S. Navy Instructional film on Basic Typing Methods, 1944, https://archive.org/details/basic_typing_1). This is in stark contrast to early office computer systems which were often installed on existing furniture with no or little training for users.

1. Good posture was defined and demonstrated
2. Trainees were shown how to use a chair with a firmly sprung back (lumbar) support
3. Trainees were shown to set the correct seat height – low enough to enable both feet to rest comfortably on the floor
4. The benefits of placing one foot slightly in front of the other for "proper balance" (when leaning forward) were demonstrated
5. To recognize and avoid the postural problems caused by chairs that were too high or too low
6. To sit squarely in relation to the desk with the abdomen 9–10 inches (22–125cm) from the front of the desk
7. To sit with the upper arms hanging freely by the sides and the forearms at a slight angle following the slope of the keyboard (elbows just below the level of the space bar)
8. To type with the hand and fingers in a neutral position and the wrists slightly extended.

One of the notable aspects of the training in the film is that typists weren't just trained how to type but they were trained how to adjust their workspaces and how to check that the adjustments were correct (Figure 2.10). This is in contrast to the 1980s when the use of visual display terminals in offices became widespread. Most office workers in the 1980s were never taught how to arrange their desks from the outset – let alone how to type. This may be one of the causes of the Cumulative Trauma Disorder (CTD) epidemic which afflicted office workers in many developed countries in the late 1980s and early 1990s (although psychological and social factors cannot be ruled out, see Arksey (1988) for a discussion of CTD from a sociological perspective).

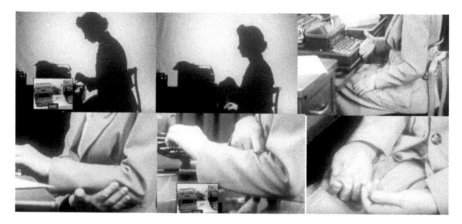

**FIGURE 2.10**  Typists' training for optimum work arrangements (L to R). Sitting too high; sitting too low; checking the keyboard distance is optimal; checking elbow height is correct; checking forearm angle; optimum hand posture for typing. (Source: U.S. Navy Instructional film on Basic Typing Methods, 1944, https://archive.org/details/basic_typing_1.)

## OFFICE LANDSCAPE CONCEPT – "BUROLANDSCHAFT"

The office landscape concept was derived from ideas about Industrial Democracy which emerged in the 1960s (Figure 2.11). There were no private offices, there was an avoidance of status symbols and a rejection of "factory-like" arrangements of furniture in favor of a more "organic" approach. Landscaping meant that physical layout was no longer used to differentiate status – this was perceived as a disadvantage for management. The open-plan layout was intended to improve communication and facilitate workflow but office staff complained of noise, distracting movement of people and lack of privacy. As the ideology underlying the open-plan office was replaced by more function-oriented thinking and increased competitive pressure was brought to bear on organizations, these ideas were increasingly challenged.

## SEDENTARY WORK IN THE COMPUTERIZED OFFICE

The 1970s and 1980s saw the widespread computerization of office work which soon led to changes in office design – in particular greater subdivision of spaces and use of paneling and screens to provide greater control of the work environment of the seated computer operators (Figure 2.12). Visual display terminals at the time used screens based on cathode ray tubes. These terminals were heavy and bulky

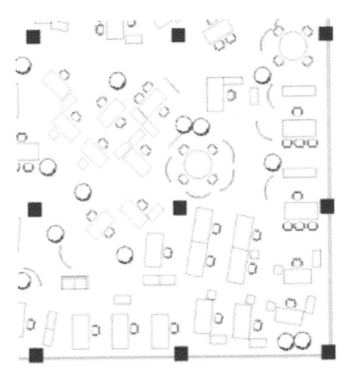

**FIGURE 2.11**   Landscape office layout 1970s with workstations arranged in a more naturalistic style interspersed with plants and other features. (Source: image courtesy of WikiMedia Commons.

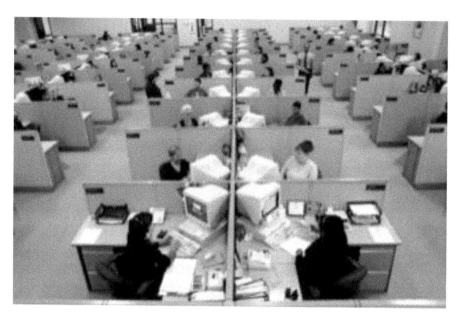

**FIGURE 2.12** Modular office with cubicles – the much maligned "cubicle farm". The introduction of computers into offices in the late 1970s to 1980s occurred rapidly and gave impetus to new designs of offices. However, the underlying philosophy and economic drivers were much the same as before and the need for workers to sit was unquestioned. Only the design of chairs changed to meet the requirements of viewing vertical screens instead of reading and writing on flat desks. Bullpen and modular office layouts are still common 40 years later. (Source: image courtesy of K2 Space, London, hello@k2-space.co.uk.)

and there was a need for built-in "systems" furniture to support the heavy screens and hide all the cabling needed to power them. Since almost all that needed to be done, was done at the computer, workers seated in modular workspaces were easy to supervise. Some of the key characteristics of these offices were:

1. Seated workstations were the norm
2. Maximizing space utilization was a main driver of the office design
3. Same overall management philosophy as before – only the technology was different.

These so-called "bullpen" offices of the 1970s were the electronic offspring of the paperwork factories at the turn of the 20th century and followed the same basic management philosophy. Even today, despite 40 years of hardware and software development, bullpen layouts can still be found.

It was with the introduction of computers into the office, that office work became increasingly sedentary – since almost all that needed to be done and all that was needed to do it were accessed from the visual display terminal. This, as we shall see in the following chapters, combined with demographic and other changes in society to create serious health problems.

## KEY POINTS

1. Are centralized systems still necessary, cost-effective or the most efficient option? We need to look at the organizational structure, and the needs of different workgroups to decide.

2. 20th-century offices were designed with chairs, desks and sedentary work to meet a requirement. Chairs, fixed desks and sedentary work were solutions to control the flow and processing of paperwork in support of the business. In the 21st-century offices, consider whether this requirement still exists when the "paperwork" is digital and work "flows" through the internet.

3. Today office workers use laptops and smartphones to work and communicate. Work flows via intranets and the internet, bringing into question the 20th-century view of office work in which "everyone knew their place and sat in it" and the idea that physical proximity and removal of physical barriers is needed for communication. In many offices today, physical barriers are no longer barriers to formal communication and work flow.

4. The training tips from the 1944 U.S. Navy instructional film are valid and are forerunners to the advice given in modern standards such as ANSI/HFEs 100-2007 https://ergoweb.com/new-ansihfes-standard-for-computer-workstations-a-milestone/. Two key points that are still relevant today, particularly in relation to the use of sit-stand workstations are that:

    a. The need to train typists in workstation ergonomics was formally recognized by management and incorporated into a proper training program.

    b. The correct guidance was identified, tested and endorsed by experts and incorporated into the training at an early stage in the typists' careers.

5. Should we be teaching 21st-century office workers how to be more active when working and how to adjust new furniture such as sit-stand desks?

    a. Key points for sedentary computer work:

        i. Desk height to be adjusted so that the feet rest firmly on the floor with no pressure under the thighs.

        ii. Seat depth shorter than the length of the thigh to prevent the seat digging into the back of the knee when using the lumbar support.

        iii. Space between the back of the seat and the backrest to allow the lumbar support to function ("sacral space").

        iv. Keyboard and mouse within the "zone of convenient reach" – no more than 40cm in front of the body.

        v. Screen height no higher than eye height when sitting up straight.

        vi. Keyboard at the same height as the elbows.

        vii. Wrist rests, footrests and document holders to be provided, as required.

    b. Key points for standing computer work:

        i. Free space and no obstructions under the desk to allow for changes in foot position.

        ii. Screen at an appropriate distance from the front of the desk to allow for comfortable viewing (about 70cm).

iii. Keyboard height at approximately elbow height when arms hang comfortably at the side (Figure 2.13).
iv. Keyboard and mouse within the "zone of convenient reach" – no more than 40cm in front of the body.
v. Screen height no higher than eye height when standing up straight, no lower than 30 degrees below the line of sight (Figure 2.14).
vi. Wrists rests, footrests and document holders to be provided, as required.

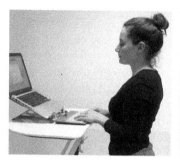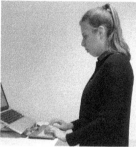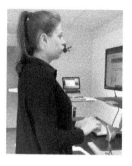

**FIGURE 2.13** Keyboard too high (wrists slightly flexed); keyboard too low (wrists extended); keyboard correct height (wrists slightly extended, in the mid-range of flexion/extension).

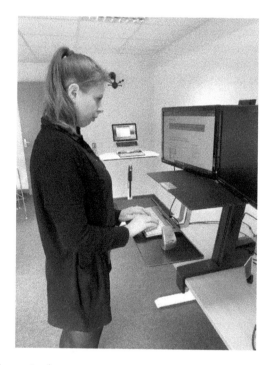

**FIGURE 2.14** Screen too low.

# 3 Are We Built to Sit?

## *Sitting as a Problem*

"Our chairs, almost without exception are designed more for the eye than the back."

**H. Staffel (quoted in Akerblom, 1954)**

Even as sedentary work became the norm in many workplaces in the 20th century, concerns were raised about the effects of sitting on the health of the workforce and the design of chairs started to be criticized.

Akerblom traced the conception of "sitting up straight" to the Ancient Egyptians. Sculptures of the Pharaohs typically depict them seated with an angle of 90 degrees between the trunk and the thighs (the "90-degree sitting posture" in Figure 3.1).

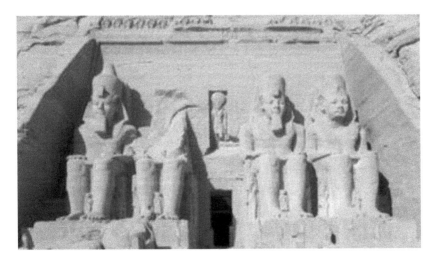

**FIGURE 3.1** Ramesses II seated on his throne at the temple of Abu Simbel. The angle between the trunk and the thighs is about 90 degrees. Sculptures such as these were made to emphasize the power and prestige of the subject. Chair designers were influenced by such art for many years until research demonstrated that the posture is effortful to maintain for any length of time and is impractical as a basis for seated work. (Source: courtesy of Pixabay.)

According to Fahrni (1966) the upright sitting posture served a cultural purpose – a mark of superiority – rather than an a practical purpose, yet it influenced chair designers for many years.

In pre-industrial Europe, even in lowly dwellings, the head of the household sat on a low stool while others sat on the floor. Medieval thrones were designed with the same cultural considerations in mind – the ruler sat above all others. In the Roman Empire, stools were reserved for magistrates and chairs with backs ("Cathedra") for ladies. Etiquette prescribed who sat on chairs and who stood or sat on the floor. The addition of a backrest to stools marked the descent of the chair down the social scale and stools without backrests were only used in specialized occupations (e.g., by milkmaids) or for special purposes (e.g., at a dressing table). The fundamental design of chairs changed little over 4000 years, although integral upholstery appeared during the Renaissance.

Thus, a conception of sitting that was initially only used to denote prestige and power descended through Western society permeating social and working life. Whereas the Ancient Romans reclined on couches while dining, their descendants in Renaissance Italy dined at table while sitting on their newly upholstered chairs. Similar chairs found their way into offices during the Industrial Revolution. Figure 3.2 depicts the conception of correct sitting used by chair designers since the

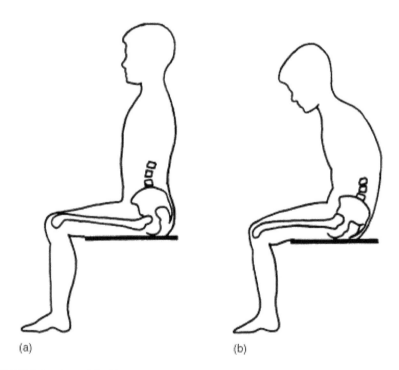

(a)                                        (b)

**FIGURE 3.2** A model of "correct sitting" that influenced furniture designers in the 19th and 20th centuries. While useful to define optimum furniture dimensions to suit a wide range of users, the posture itself is uncomfortable to maintain for long periods. The reality is that most people soon tend to slump forwards over the desk.

19th century and until recently in international standards, in the training of designers and in teaching people to sit "correctly". Most people are unable to sit comfortably this way and, when writing for example, soon slump over the desk.

Staffel (1884) recognized the importance of lumbar supports and attempted to
design a workspace to accommodate lumbar support and an upright sitting posture (Figure 3.3). Victorian designers recognized that users would not be able to sit
upright against a backrest if the head was flexed forwards to look at a flat desk. This
is why tilting work surfaces and bookstands were fitted to encourage an upright sitting posture and use of the lumbar support.

During the 1950s, it started to become clear that sitting on chairs all day was
causing problems for many people and it was J.J. Keegan (1953), an orthopedic
surgeon, who in 1953 made the first real objections to the upright sitting posture following clinical observations of thousands of low-back sufferers. After taking X-rays
of the spine and pelvis of people adopting different postures, Keegan concluded that
the requirement to sit up straight all day was unattainable for most people. Most
soon adopt a slumped posture, with the lumbar discs "wedged" posteriorly placing
pressure on nerve roots and ligaments causing pain (Figure 3.4).

Most people are unable to sit up straight with the trunk at 90 degrees to the thighs
because they can't flex the hip joints by 90 degrees. Instead, the hip joints flex by
about 60 degrees and the pelvis tips back by about 30 degrees causing the lumbar

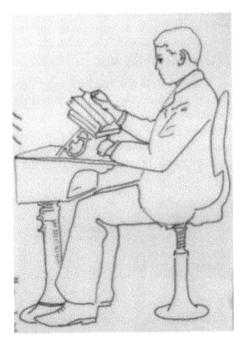

**FIGURE 3.3** Early attempts to specify the design of comfortable work chairs. The
Victorians solved the problem of slumping over the desk by incorporating worksurfaces that
tilted towards the sitter. In the early 20th century, designers began to incorporate lumbar
supports to enable sitters to recline comfortably. (Source: redrawn from Zacharow, 1988.)

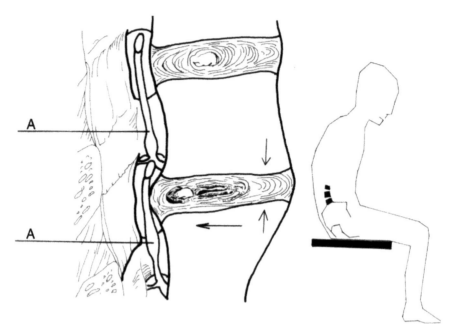

A

A

**FIGURE 3.4**   Sitting at a desk in a slumped posture causes the lumbar intervertebral discs to be "wedged" by pressure from the vertebra above (like cracking a nut in a nutcracker). This causes the fluid center of the disc to protrude posteriorly and is a source of pain in people with symptomatic lumbar discs. (Source: Bridger (2018), with permission.)

spine (in the lower part of the back) to flex resulting in a "slumped" sitting posture. The more you have to flex your hips, the more the pelvis tips back and the more rounded becomes the lower part of the spine (Figure 3.5).

Keegan demonstrated why people with symptomatic lumbar discs found sedentary work difficult and concluded that the "resting position" of the lumbar spine was when there was an angle of about 135 degrees between the trunk and the thighs.

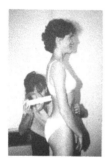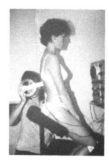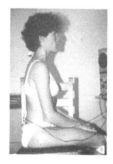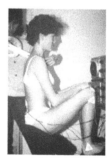

**FIGURE 3.5**   Sitting is different from standing. When we sit down, the tension in the muscles that hold the spine and pelvis in place changes. Even in healthy young people, the pelvis tips back and the spine flattens.

Keegan concluded that chairs should enable users to recline against backrests, rather than try to sit up straight. Keegan's ideas were confirmed independently by other researchers (e.g., Bridger et al., 1992a).

Probably the most dramatic example of the body in its true resting posture is shown in Figure 3.6, the posture adopted by an astronaut in space in weightless conditions with no external forces acting on the body. Under these conditions, the posture of the joints is determined by the elasticity of the ligaments and tendons around the joints and by muscle tone. In this posture, the joints are free to move in all directions. Many readers will recognize the posture in Figure 3.6 – we often wake up lying on our side in a similar position.

Despite the evidence that was accumulating that we are *not* built to sit on chairs all day, chair designers continued to develop the conventional seating models throughout the 1950s and 1960s. Useful advances were made in chair design, cushioning and contouring, for example, and the realization that although chairs with very deep seats (front to back) look more comfortable, they are not. Support is only needed under the seat bones ("ischial tuberosities") and can be harmful if there is too much pressure under the thighs such that it restricts blood flow in the soft tissues of the legs.

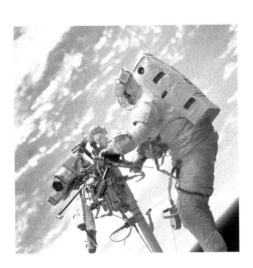
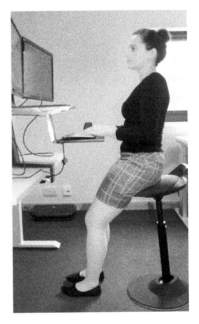

**FIGURE 3.6**   The human body in "neutral." An astronaut in space. With no external forces acting on the body, only internal forces due to the elasticity of ligaments and muscles influence posture. This posture is approximated when we recline in a chair, "perch" on the edge of a table, or use a "perch" stool to work at a standing desk. (Source: image courtesy of Pixabay.)

## SITTING AS A PROBLEM RATHER THAN A SOLUTION

By the early 1970s, it had become clear that we are *not* built to sit all day. Habitual daily activities influence the incidence of disease and mechanical strain on the spine is greater when sitting that when standing (Figure 3.7). Furthermore, evidence was emerging that backache is more common in people who sit all day than in those who combine standing and sitting (Magora, 1972). More recently, Vink et al. (2009) found that people reported less musculoskeletal pain, including backache, when using sit-stand workstations where they could sit, stand or semi-stand at will, as opposed to traditional chairs and desks.

## TACKLING "HOMO SEDENS" IN THE OFFICE

The introduction of computers into the office from the 1970s onwards brought a major change – instead of the reading and writing on documents on a flat desk, office workers stared at near-vertical computer screens. Initially, there were few fundamental changes to the design of office chairs, but it was not long after the

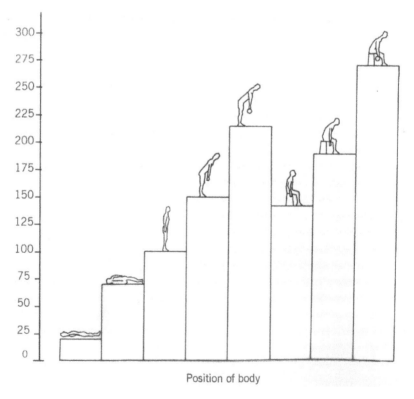

Position of body

**FIGURE 3.7**   The load on the lumbar discs in different positions of the body. Disc pressure, which is strongly associated with the occurrence of back pain, is higher in most sitting postures than it is when standing. Backache in sedentary workers may be relieved by intermittent standing. (Source: redrawn from Nachemson, 1966.)

widespread introduction of computers in offices that new concepts in chair design started to emerge.

New chairs designs were needed to accommodate the change in posture from leaning forwards and looking down at a flat desk to leaning back and looking straight ahead at a computer screen. One of the new ideas was championed by Dr. A.C. Mandal (1987), who in 1982 observed that over the preceding 100 years, the populations of industrialized countries had grown taller, while the height of desks had been reduced! Mandal proposed that instead of sitting on chairs with our thighs at 90 degrees to our trunks and parallel to the floor, we should work at higher desks on chairs designed for the purpose (Figure 3.8). Note the sloping desktop, dating from Strasser's (1913) time, was retained but the high desk enabled users to sit with a larger angle between the trunk and the legs similar to the posture of the astronaut in Figure 3.6.

Figure 3.9 shows tracing from X-rays taken from the side of a person (the author) in a standing position, sitting at a high desk in the manner proposed by Mandal and in the 90-degree position of Ramases II. In standing, the concave curve in the lower back is apparent (the lumbar lordosis). In the 90-degree posture it is absent and at the high desk some of the curvature is retained, with the spine supporting the mass of the upper body without "wedging" the lumbar discs in the manner observed by Keegan. Mandal also recognized that a tilted work surface would encourage an upright sitting posture because it would reduce the need to flex the neck or lean forwards.

*The high desk and chair proposed by Mandal clearly had many advantages over conventional desks and chairs. One, of course, which does not appear to have been discussed at the time, was that one might also stand and work at the high desk with its sloping work surface in the manner of the Victorian standing desk in Figure 2.3. That this was not discussed reflects the views of the time that office work was sedentary and that standing was unhealthy.*

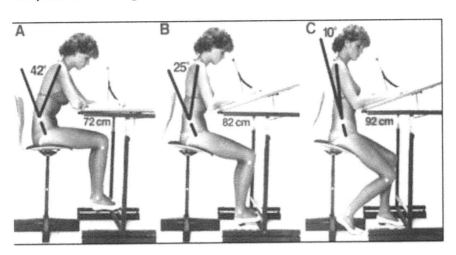

**FIGURE 3.8**   High desks and sloping seats. Dr. A.C. Mandal's proposal for a new approach to seating in the 1980s. (Source: Mandal (1987), courtesy of Dr. A.C. Mandal.)

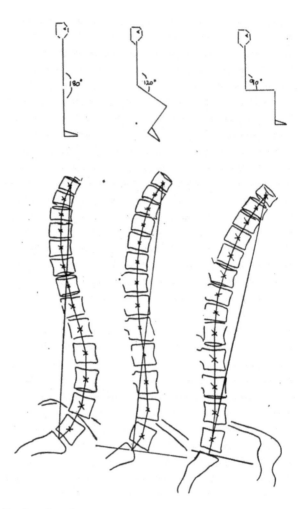

**FIGURE 3.9**    Tracings from X-rays of the spine from left to right: standing, sitting on a high chair, sitting on a conventional chair. Note progressive loss of the lumbar curve.

At the same time, a radical new seating concept emerged – the "Balans Chair" (Figure 3.10).

Both the Balans Chair and the seat proposed by Mandal were designed to enable users to sit with an upright trunk and with an angle between the trunk and the thighs of 115 degrees or greater. Two main differences are that when kneeling on the Balans chair the base of support is much larger than any conventional seat and the posture is more stable. A second difference is that the knees are flexed thereby shortening the hamstring muscles and placing the pelvis and spine close to their neutral positions (Bridger et al., 1992a).

Despite the obvious advantages of these concepts, they did not lead to a new generation of office chairs to replace conventional chairs and desks in the newly computerized offices of the 1980s (possibly because Mandal's proposal, in particular,

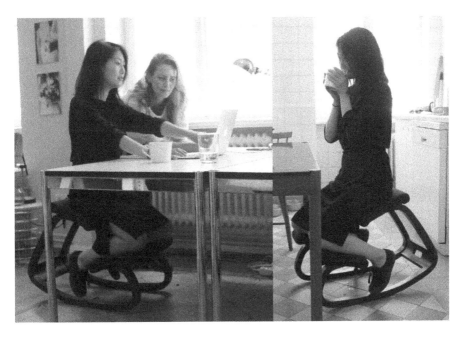

**FIGURE 3.10** "Kneeling Chair" based on the "Balans" Chair invented in 1979 by Hans Christian Mengshoel. This design has a curved base enabling a slight rocking motion while seated. (Source: photos courtesy of Back in Action – The Back Shop, London, United Kingdom.)

required replacing the desks as well as the chairs). However, with the development of new construction materials for chairs (such as carbon reinforced plastic), improved chairs for use at conventional desks soon appeared such as that in Figure 3.11.

These chairs had high backrests with lower (lumbar) and upper back support and used new materials such that the backrest "followed" the user when reclining or sitting up straight. The space between the seat and the lumbar support enabled the lumbar support to engage the lumbar spine in a variety of postures. Essentially these chairs brought an end to the concept of the 90-degree sitting posture, enabling users to recline with an angle between the trunk and the thighs closer to Keegan's recommended 115–135 degrees.

A key feature of the new computer chairs was that they readily supported a wider variety of sitting postures, including the more "open" sitting posture recommended by Mandal and Keegan. Reclining postures were achieved by incorporating a flexible backrest to support the upper back while the contour of the backrest provided lumbar support. A space between the seat and the backrest enabled the buttocks to protrude posteriorly and the lumbar support used the lumbar spine as a lever to keep the pelvis tilted forwards thereby retaining some of the lumbar lordosis. The compressive load on the spine was reduced when reclining, since the backrest bore some of the weight of the upper body and head.

Many large organizations invested in the new furniture. However, not all provided their employees with training on how to get the best out of their new chairs.

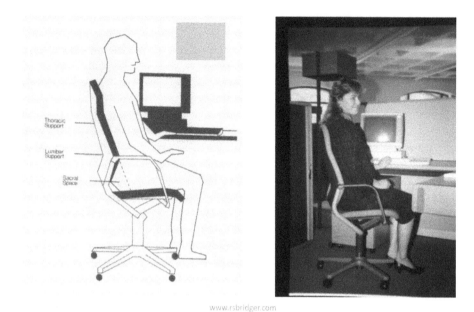

**FIGURE 3.11**   1980s computer chair – note the high, flexible backrest to enable the user to recline while working at a terminal. The base of the backrest provides space for the buttocks to preserve the "S"-shape of the spine. Excellent biomechanics but the energy expenditure is little different from staying in bed all day.

The need to standardize on one type of chair for the organization sometimes resulted in chairs being purchased with seats that were too deep for short females. Recall that chair designers of the early 20th century recognized that typists, in those days typists were predominantly female, needed smaller chairs than managers, predominantly male. Early typists chairs, in particular, had shallow seats (from front to back) so that even short users could sit back in the seat to engage the backrest without the front of the seat digging into the back of the knee. Standardizing on chairs for the new computerized offices sometimes resulted in purchase of chairs that were too deep and shorter computer users spent their days "perched" on the front edge of the seat.

Despite these limitations, the new computer chairs had several advantages over their predecessors: users could look straight ahead at the screen when reclining; the backrest supported some of the weight of the trunk and reduced pressure on the intervertebral discs; the spine retained its more natural "S" shape when reclining with a lumbar support; by means of springs or other means, the backrest remained in contact with the trunk when the user changed posture.

These chairs were comfortable and were an advance on their predecessors but there was one main disadvantage – a physiological one. *In terms of energy expenditure, spending the day reclining on an office chair does not use much more energy than spending the day in bed.*

## SITTING AND PHYSICAL INACTIVITY

At the time of its introduction, new office furniture (sometimes called "Systems Furniture") brought significant improvements in office workstation design. However, what was not apparent at the time, was that work in the newly computerized offices had become even less physically demanding than that in the paperwork factories of the past. For most of the 20th century, prior to the introduction of computers into offices, office work was rarely completely sedentary. Because paper flowed through the office, employees often had to physically transport the paper from their desks to other locations. Records were stored in filing cabinets or records offices, rather than electronic databases and employees would have to leave their desks to refer to these throughout the day. Prior to the debut of the electronic office, sedentary work in offices was interspersed with walking. Since the large-scale introduction of computers into offices, beginning in the 1970s and becoming almost universal by the late 1980s, office work had become increasingly sedentary with employees "tied" to their computers spending most of the day sitting.

*So, it would seem that the biomechanical solutions to the problems of sedentary work have exacerbated the physiological problem of a lack of physical activity. The more comfortable the chair and the more we can recline on it, the more inactive we are.*

With the demographic changes of the 21st century in many countries, the problem of "Homo Sedens," the seated man, took on a new meaning and new solutions were required.

As we will see in the next chapter, it was not only sitting at work that was the problem, but *sedentarism*, the sedentary lifestyles of many in the population both at work and at home and the health problems that developed in the population as a result.

## KEY POINTS

1. Are we built to sit? Yes, but not on chairs, not in the 90-degree sitting posture and not for eight hours per day.
2. Backache, in those susceptible to it, is often related to compression of the spine and, in particular, compression of the intervertebral discs. The disc pressure is greater in sitting than in standing, which may explain why people with symptomatic lumbar discs experience pain more frequently when sitting rather than standing and why they might benefit from standing to work at a desk, rather than sitting all day.
3. As a general rule, changing one's posture throughout the day is beneficial for a variety of reasons – avoidance of back pain and, as we shall see later, improvements in blood circulation and metabolism.
4. Typists in the 20th century were sometimes trained how to sit down on a chair to obtain maximum lumbar support (Figure 3.12):
   a. Sit on the front edge of the seat
   b. Lean forward from the hip
   c. Slide the buttocks to the back of the seat
   d. Straighten up against the backrest.

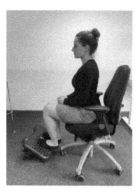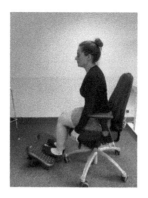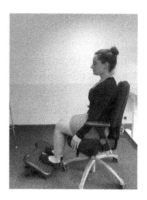

**FIGURE 3.12**   Maximizing lumbar support. Sit down on the front edge of the chair, lean forwards from the hip, slide back and lean into the backrest.

5. Old conceptions of efficiency, which saw sedentary work as the norm may have been the best solution in the paperwork factories of the 20th century. Even then, most workers were never completely sedentary and would leave their desks to access filing cabinets and storerooms, to collect mail and so on. With the advent of the computerized office, employees were increasingly tied to their desks all day with no reason to leave. There are now valid reasons for questioning the value of sedentary work as the standard model, both in terms of productivity and in terms of employee health.

6. Taken together the evidence suggests that there is no "best" way of sitting that is appropriate for everyone. Despite the efforts of designers to standardize sedentary office work, the evidence has accumulated that there is no "one size fits all" solution and that movement should be designed into office work.

7. As is described in more detail in the next chapter, sitting at a computer all day on a well-designed office chair is barely more active than staying in bed all day.

# 4 Physical Activity in Everyday Life

## *Demographic Change in the 21st Century*

Recognition of the role of exercise in health is changing as robots and auto-mation now perform most of the laborious tasks that used to be done by muscle power. A cartoon in an American newspaper recently quipped, "Time was when most men who finished a day's work needed rest. Now they need exercise!"

**Paffenbarger et al. (1984)**

Many adults are physically inactive nowadays. An inactive lifestyle is defined as not engaging in physical activity or exercise in the last 30 days. In the USA in 2017, 19.2 percent and 19.5 percent of adults in the states of Washington and Colorado were physically inactive compared to 33.2 percent and 34.4 percent in the states of Mississippi and Kentucky (Robert Wood Johnson Foundation, 2018). Even in the most "active" states, a large number of people were inactive. This is a recent phe-nomenon and has major implications for the health of the workforce and the associ-ated costs of ill health including medical costs and loss of productivity.

At the turn of the 20th century when the Larkin Building was built, 30.9 per-cent of the U.S. workforce worked in agriculture and about 38.9 percent worked in manufacturing and associated trades. In 2015 the percentages were 0.7 percent for agriculture and 20.2 percent for manufacturing. Similarly, the percentage of pro-fessional, technical and service workers has increased from 20.9 percent to 56.6 percent. The physical demands of the working life of a large percentage of the popu-lation have diminished over the last 100 years, as have the physical demands of private life – years ago, many workers walked to work and had few labor-saving devices at home.

## SEDENTARY WORK IS PHYSICALLY UNDEMANDING

We saw earlier that a great deal of attention was paid to the design of chairs when offices were computerized in the 1970s and 1980s. In terms of body mechanics, many of the new seats were excellent. However, whereas in old "pencil and paper" offices, employees had to leave their desks throughout the day to visit filing cabinets, storerooms, record offices, libraries and so on, the newly computerized offices saw employees reclining in computer chairs all day long. *The energy cost and metabolic effect of this activity is little different from spending all day in bed.*

It is now well established that physical inactivity is harmful and that too many people spend too much time sitting at work, sitting while commuting to and from work and sitting at home (Straker and Mathiassen, 2009).

## PHYSICAL INACTIVITY AND MORTALITY

A study was carried out in Taiwan by Wen et al. (2011) who analyzed life expectancy in 416,175 healthy people in relation to self-reported lifestyle and other risk factors for mortality. They found a strong relationship between physical inactivity in leisure time and increased mortality due to heart disease, diabetes, and cancer in the following years.

Wen et al. (2011) asked people to report their daily leisure physical activity and classified the reported activity levels as follows:

1. Light activity such as walking (2.5 METS)
2. Moderate activity such as brisk walking (4.5 METS)
3. Medium vigorous activity such as jogging (6.5 METS)
4. High-vigorous activity such as running (8.5 METS).

The "MET" (metabolic equivalent) is a unit of physical activity that indicates the intensity of the activity. One MET is equivalent to the resting metabolic rate (the energy required to maintain all the bodily processes essential for life when completely relaxed and at rest). So, watching television has a value of one MET whereas sleeping has a value of 0.9 METs. Sedentary office work (e.g., when using a keyboard and looking at a screen) has a value of about 1.5 METS or lower. Standing still has a MET value of 1.59 METS (Mansoubi et al., 2015). Walking slowly has a value of 2 METS.

Participants in the study also reported the number of hours per week they engaged in different activities and the activity was quantified as "MET hours" per week (the sum of the number of hours per week spent in activities at different MET levels). So, for example, someone reporting jogging (6.5 METS) for three hours per week would score 19.5 MET hours of jogging activity (three hours at 6.5 METS). The participants were then placed into one of five physical activity categories: inactive (<3.75 MET hours), low (3.75–7.49 MET hours), medium (7.50–16.49 MET hours), high (16.50–25.49 MET hours), or very high (≥25.50 MET hours). They were also split into two groups on the basis of whether some or all of the exercise they engaged in every week was vigorous.

The participants were followed for an average of 8.05 years after reporting their physical activity levels and "all-cause mortality" (whether any of them died for any reason) was recorded. The data were analyzed to determine whether leisure-time physical activity was related to subsequent mortality, taking into account factors such as pre-existing medical conditions, smoking and job demands.

When compared with individuals in the *inactive* group, those in the low-volume activity group had a lower risk of all-cause mortality, irrespective of their sex, age, or health status, or whether or not they smoked, drank, or had pre-existing cardiovascular disease risk. So, even light exercise for an hour per week is beneficial. Vigorous-intensity exercise yielded similar or greater health benefits in terms of all-cause mortality reduction than did moderate-intensity exercise at the same amount of activity or at the next higher amount of physical activity. Vigorous activities tend to have higher MET values than less demanding activities, so the benefits of being physically active can be achieved in fewer hours per week with vigorous activity.

One of the most interesting findings in this study is that even low levels of physical activity are better than no activity at all. People in the low-volume physical activity group (only exercising about 15 minutes per day) had a 14 percent reduction in mortality and three-year increased life expectancy compared to those who were inactive. Every additional 15 minutes of exercise per day increased life expectancy by 4 percent!

*How can such a small increase in physical activity bring such large benefits?*

As is explained below, it is not only the case that exercise is beneficical for health – it is the *lack* of physical activity that is *harmful in itself.*

## PHYSICAL INACTIVITY IS HARMFUL

The benefits of a physically active lifestyle are well established. Physical inactivity is estimated to account for 6 percent of global deaths. The World Health Organization recommends that adults participate in at least 150 minutes of (at least) moderate-intensity physical activity throughout the week to reduce the risk of chronic disease, including cardiovascular disease, Type 2 diabetes and certain cancers. Much modern work in offices is mentally demanding and physically undemanding. As we will see shortly, it is the combination of the two that is particularly hazardous to health.

## BENEFITS OF EXERCISE

Exercise is beneficial – not just because it "burns calories" but because it helps maintain a healthy metabolism. One of the more interesting sources of evidence in support of this idea is research on bed-rest that was carried in support of the NASA space program due to concerns about the health of astronauts living in weightless conditions (Figure 4.1). A brief look at studies of bed-rest and why physical inactivity is harmful to the health of otherwise healthy people is useful if we are to understand why sitting all day might be harmful.

According to Bergouignan et al. (2011) bed-rest studies indicate that physical inactivity is a main cause of *metabolic inflexibility.*

Metabolic inflexibility has four components.

*Insulin resistance*: The body becomes less sensitive to insulin. Insulin is a hormone that is released from the pancreas – normally when blood glucose levels rise after a meal. Insulin enables target tissues such as the skeletal muscles and the liver to take up glucose from the blood and either store it for later use or use it for energy. The amount of glucose in the blood then falls to safe levels (high levels of glucose in the blood can damage nerves, blood vessels and organs).

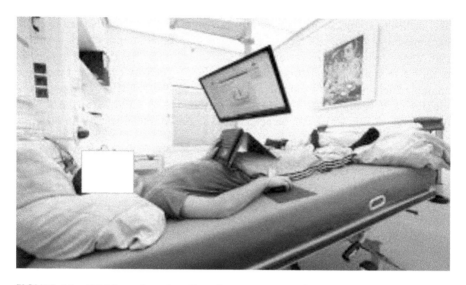

**FIGURE 4.1**   NASA conducted studies of astronauts to understand the effects of physical inactivity on otherwise healthy people. These "bed-rest" studies showed that bed-rest causes "metabolic inflexibility" – including a reduced ability to metabolize fat. Note that reclining in an office chair for eight hours is little more physically demanding than staying in bed all day.

The effect of insulin resistance is that the target tissues no longer respond to insulin as they should, glucose is not taken up from the blood and blood glucose levels remain elevated. In the long term, elevated blood glucose levels can cause a variety of health problems including high blood pressure.

*Changes in blood cholesterol*: Blood triglyceride levels increase, LDL ("bad") cholesterol levels increase; HDL ("good") cholesterol levels decrease.

*Lowered insulin sensitivity in the muscles*: Physical inactivity promotes fat storage. Physical inactivity shunts the delivery of lipids in the blood plasma away from the muscles (where it would be used as an energy source) to adipose tissue (where it is stored as fat). In other words, instead of the lipids being used for energy, they are stored as fat.

*A shift in substrate use towards glucose*: Human skeletal muscles normally use fatty acids as the "default" source of energy. In healthy people, "muscles burn fat." Metabolic inflexibility impairs the capacity to use fatty acids as an energy source when the availability of fatty acids increases. In all bed-rest studies, a shift in fuel metabolism is observed in favor of carbohydrate oxidation and to the detriment of lipid oxidation.

According to the bed-rest studies, then, physical inactivity reduces the capacity of the body to use fat as an energy source; causes muscle loss; and causes resistance to insulin, elevated blood sugar levels, and elevated levels of triglycerides and cholesterol.

As might be expected from the laboratory research described above, similar harmful effects of physical inactivity have been found in studies of the general population over longer time periods. Katzmarzyk et al. (2009) followed 1543 Canadian adults over 15 years. All were free of Type II diabetes at the beginning. At the end of the study 5 percent had developed diabetes. Being overweight at the beginning of the study and having a low level of physical activity predicted the development of diabetes.

## OVERWEIGHT, OBESITY AND TYPE II DIABETES

Over the last 70 years, there has been a marked increase in the number of overweight and obese people in the population. Parikh et al. (2007) reported that, whereas in the 1950s 21.8 percent of men in the USA were overweight and 5.8 percent were obese, by 2000 35.2 percent were overweight and 14.8 percent were obese. For women, 15 percent were overweight and 3.9 percent obese in the 1950s, compared to 33.1 percent and 14 percent by 2000.

*Overweight and obesity is not new and the U.S. data shows a clear trend over five decades, rather than a sudden increase.*

About 40 percent of adults in the USA were obese in 2015–2016, up from 34 percent in 2007–2008 (Hales, 2018). Similar trends have been observed in other developed countries such as the United Kingdom and Australia.

There has also been a corresponding increase in the prevalence of Type II diabetes since the 1950s. According to the Center for Disease Control in the USA (CDC, 2017), in 1958 0.93 percent of the U.S. population had diabetes compared with 7.4 percent in 2015. In 2015, 23.4 million people in the USA had been diagnosed with diabetes, compared to only 1.6 million in 1958.

## PHYSICAL INACTIVITY AT WORK

Clearly, there are several factors underlying the trend in obesity. According to the U.S. Bureau of Labor Statistics, in 1915, food and alcohol consumption accounted for 30 percent of total personal spending compared to about 16 percent today – food is a lot more affordable nowadays.

Diet is one of the main contributors to obesity and physical inactivity is another.

Over the last 50 years, industries in many developed countries have introduced increased mechanization and automation and the service sector of their economies has increased in size. In the decade after World War II, 70 percent of the British workforce were in some kind of manual labor. Most women worked only part-time or at home where labor-saving devices were few and housework was more physically demanding (for a fascinating insight into the demands of housework, prior to the advent of modern labor-saving devices, see Grandjean, 1973).

Much of the work in modern service industries is physically undemanding. Sedentary office work has an activity level of about 1.5 METS. So, an office worker on a 40-hour working week would have a work activity level of about 60 MET hours. For illustrative purposes, we can compare the weekly activity level of an office worker with that of a housewife in the 1950s (Figure 4.2).

For simplicity, let's assume that neither did any exercise outside of work, and confine our comparison to a working week of 40 hours (in fact, the housewife probably

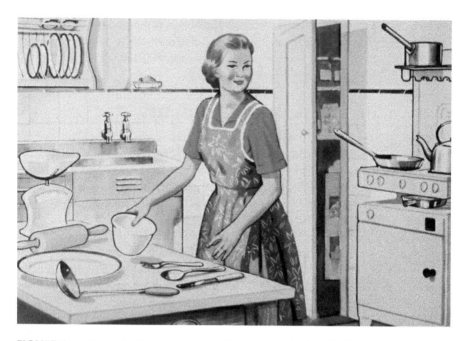

**FIGURE 4.2**   Trends in Physical Activity. Physical activity in daily life has reduced since the introduction of labor-saving devices. An average housewife in the 1950s would spend a considerable part of every day standing while engaged in light to moderate manual work of 2–5 METS. To match this over a working week, a sedentary office worker would need to add ten or more hours of aerobics after work! (Source: image from Pixabay.)

worked much longer than this). Assuming the housewife had minimal labor saving devices, her working week might have looked something like this:

So, the housewife's activity level for the 40-hour working week is 124.4 MET hours compared to 60 MET hours for the modern office worker. This is a difference of 64.4 MET hours. To be as physically active as a 1950s housewife, the office

**TABLE 4.1**

| Activity | Activity Level METS | Hours/Week |
|---|:---:|:---:|
| General Cleaning | 3.5 | 6 |
| Cooking | 2.5 | 10 |
| Washing dishes | 2.1 | 3 |
| Washing floor | 3.3 | 2 |
| Ironing | 2.0 | 4 |
| Making beds | 4.0 | 2 |
| Pushing child's chair | 4.0 | 3 |
| Carrying (shopping/infant) | 4.5 | 2 |
| Walking up/downstairs | 4.0 | 1 |
| Cleaning/Sweeping | 3.5 | 2 |
| Playing with children | 3.5 | 5 |

worker would then have to exercise more after work – the equivalent of spending ten hours per week in an aerobics class (about 6 METS) or five hours per week playing squash (about 12 METS)!

## IS SITTING THE NEW SMOKING?

Greer et al. (2015) found that men who sat for four to eight hours or more than eight hours per day had 65 percent and 76 percent greater risk of developing *metabolic syndrome* than those less sedentary. This is important because metabolic syndrome is a precursor to Type II diabetes where the body becomes insensitive to insulin and there is a risk of chronically elevated blood glucose levels causing damage to arteries and high blood pressure. The International Diabetes Federation defines metabolic syndrome as follows:

> The metabolic syndrome is a cluster of the most dangerous heart attack risk factors: diabetes and raised fasting plasma glucose, abdominal obesity, high cholesterol and high blood pressure. It is estimated that around 20–25 per cent of the world's adult population have the metabolic syndrome and they are twice as likely to die from and three times as likely to have a heart attack or stroke compared with people without the syndrome.
>
> In addition, people with metabolic syndrome have a five-fold greater risk of developing type 2 diabetes. They would add to the 230 million people worldwide who already have diabetes one of the most common chronic diseases worldwide and the fourth or fifth leading cause of death in the developed world. The clustering of cardiovascular disease (CVD) risk factors that typifies the metabolic syndrome is now considered to be the driving force for a new CVD (cardiovascular disease) epidemic.
>
> **(Alberti et al., 2006)**

The harmful effects of a sedentary lifestyle remained when physical activity and cardio-respiratory fitness were controlled for in the analysis (and vice versa). In other words, those who sat for long periods each day were more likely to develop metabolic syndrome than those who sat less, even if they were physically fit and active. At the same time, people who were more active and had better cardiovascular fitness were less likely to develop metabolic syndrome even if they were sedentary. It is important to note that these findings indicate that the increased risk of metabolic syndrome in those who spent a lot of time sitting was not because these individuals were unfit or had cardiovascular problems which caused the sedentary lifestyle. *It was because they spent a lot of time sitting.* Or, to put it another way, people are more likely to be active when they are not sitting down! So, sedentary behavior and a lack of physical fitness are independent risk factors for metabolic syndrome.

In the same way that physically fit tobacco smokers are more at risk of health problems than physically fit non-smokers, physically fit people who sit a lot are more at risk of health problems than physically fit people who sit less. This may explain why some have said that sitting is the "new smoking."

## IS SITTING REALLY THE NEW SMOKING?

Not really. The author knows of no jobs where there is an occupational requirement to smoke tobacco whereas in many office jobs, employees have no option but to sit.

The health benefits of regular exercise are well understood and evidence is mounting that it is not just how much time we spend exercising that protects us, but what we do the rest of the time (when we are not exercising). Van der Ploeg et al. (2012) found further evidence for the independent relationship of sitting time with all-cause mortality. The researchers linked questionnaire data from 222,497 people aged 45 years or older to mortality data from the New South Wales Registry of Births, Deaths, and Marriages (Australia) from February 1, 2006, through December 31, 2010. The researchers recorded all-cause mortality (death for any reason in the period of the study) in relation to sitting time. The effects of sitting time on all-cause mortality were examined and other potential causes of death controlled for and ruled out (including sex, age at the time of the study, education, urban/rural residence, physical activity, body mass index, smoking status, self-rated health, and disability). Sitting time was divided into four categories: less than 4 hours per day; 4–8 hours per day; 8–11 hours per day; and greater than 11 hours per day.

During the years of follow-up (mean follow-up, 2.8 years), 5405 deaths were registered. There was an 11 percent increase in all-cause mortality for every increase in sitting time across the four categories. The association between sitting and all-cause mortality appeared consistent across the sexes, age groups, body mass index categories, and physical activity levels and across healthy participants compared with participants with pre-existing cardiovascular disease or diabetes mellitus. The authors found that prolonged sitting is a risk factor for all-cause mortality, independent of physical activity and that public health programs should focus on reducing sitting time in addition to increasing physical activity levels.

This research demonstrates that inactive participants who spent a lot of time sitting had the highest mortality rate. A strong relationship of increased sitting time to mortality persisted, even among participants with relatively high levels of physical activity. As might be expected, healthy participants had lower absolute all-cause mortality rates (dying for any reason) compared with participants with pre-existing cardiovascular disease or diabetes. Increased physical activity and reduced sitting were associated with lower death rates in both groups. High levels of sitting were associated with higher death rates even when body mass index (a measure of overweight and obesity) was controlled for (even slim "sitters" had increased risk compared to slim "non-sitters").

Wilmot et al. (2012) analyzed the findings of 18 studies looking at the links between daily sitting time, cardiovascular disease and death in a sample totaling 794,577 participants. Overall the associations between sedentary time and adverse health outcomes were strong and consistent across the studies, even when physical activity was controlled for. Again, the researchers found that the link between sedentary behavior and adverse health outcomes was largely independent of physical activity. In fact many sedentary behaviors such as TV viewing are weakly correlated with participation in moderate-to-vigorous physical activity, because people tend not to trade-off exercise with TV viewing (physically active people also watch television – there is plenty of time in any 24-hour period to engage in vigorous physical activity to reach Wen et al.'s (2011) "very active" target of 25.5 MET hours per week and still watch television in the evenings). However, sedentary time was more strongly correlated with light intensity physical activity. Therefore substituting sitting with light intensity physical activity may reduce the risk of future health problems in everyone.

So, it is probably misleading to say that sitting is the "new smoking" because the health risks of sitting and smoking are not the same. However, there is plenty of evidence to support the conclusion that the longer one sits per day, the greater the risk of diabetes and cardiovascular disease in the future. Exercise also protects against these conditions but it does so independently. In the same way, tobacco smokers who exercise may be less likely to suffer health problems than smokers that don't, but if they want to reduce the risk further they should give up smoking.

## STANDING TO WORK AT YOUR COMPUTER – WILL IT MAKE A DIFFERENCE AND HOW LONG DO YOU NEED TO STAND AT WORK?

On a typical work day, an office worker might spend about 1–2 hours eating, 2 hours seated while commuting, 7–8 hours seated at work and 3 hours watching television – maybe 14 hours in total. According to the studies reviewed in the previous section, this is well above the 11 hours of sitting per day that is the highest risk group. Spending 4 hours per day standing at work would lower the total to 10 hours sitting per day – at the boundary of the next lowest risk group. The studies imply that introducing sit-stand workstations into offices will be beneficial if office workers spend a considerable portion of the working day standing. This would be a major change for many and might lead to other problems as we shall see in the next chapter.

## IS STANDING MORE ACTIVE THAN SITTING?

From the perspective of energy consumption, standing still is barely more physically demanding than sitting and less demanding than active tasks such as playing computer games while sitting down (Mansoubi et al., 2015). This is because the human body is well designed to maintain an upright standing posture, as we saw in Chapter 1. The human spine is shaped such that the weight of the body "sits" on a column of bone and when standing still is like an inverted pendulum, exquisitely balanced by the postural muscles, swaying almost imperceptibly to maintain position (except in people who are about to faint or are drunk!).

Mansoubi et al. (2015) reported MET values for standing and sitting tasks obtained from carefully controlled laboratory studies. These researchers found that MET values for sitting tasks varied considerably, depending on the task. As expected, the MET value for watching TV was low – 1.33 METS. Standing still was slightly higher than sitting at 1.59 METS, which was lower than sitting while playing computer games (2.06 METS). MET values when walking increased from 2.17 to 3.22 METS as the speed increased from 0.2 to 1.6mph.

*So, standing still isn't much more active than sitting and can't be expected to "burn extra calories" (or not many anyway).*

A more recent experiment by Betts et al. (2018) compared the energy cost of lying down, sitting in a reclined posture and standing while watching TV. Volunteers were allowed to fidget, but had to stand on the same spot when standing. The energy expenditure was expressed as a percentage increase of the resting metabolic rate. Energy expenditure increased by 3.7 percent above the resting level when fidgeting lying down, by 6.6 percent when sitting and 19.7 percent above the resting level when standing. These increases are very small and the authors came to the following conclusions:

1. Very few people exceeded 1.5 METS when standing – which is lower than much other research would suggest.
2. Standing more at work for two hours per day would be unlikely to have any useful effect on reducing body fatness or be useful in the treatment of obesity.
3. A shift in the way work is organized at a societal level resulting in the population standing an extra hour per day might help *slow the rising trend* in obesity as long as people did not compensate in other ways (e.g., by eating more). In effect, people who become overweight or obese were not born that way and it may take years for problems to develop, so even small increases in energy expenditure may slow the rate of increase in body weight.
4. Breaking extended periods of sitting with other postures and activities may be beneficial.

So, standing is more active than sitting – but not very!

Walking is more demanding but to put this into perspective we can consider the energy costs of other daily physical activities. Walking upstairs, carrying a handbag or case weighing a few kilograms has a MET value of 5 METS – over three times as much energy as expended when standing at a desk. In practice, the implementation of sit-stand workstations on its own, or standing more at work is unlikely to increase the daily energy expenditure of office staff, whereas using the stairs instead of the escalators would bring much larger increases in energy expenditure and in a much shorter time.

But would combining standing at work with sitting bring other benefits? Yes, there is evidence that it may bring metabolic benefits as is explained below.

## BENEFITS OF NOT SITTING AFTER LUNCH

We saw earlier that blood glucose levels rise after a meal and insulin is released to lower the blood glucose level (chronically elevated blood glucose levels are harmful). The rise in blood glucose levels after lunch is exaggerated in sedentary workers (Manohar et al., 2012). Even a short walk of 15 minutes after lunch can reduce this rise in blood glucose levels by 50 percent. Buckley et al. (2014) measured blood glucose levels in people who either stood or sat for 3 hours after lunch. The rise in blood sugar levels was attenuated when people stood rather than sat and remained lower for the rest of the afternoon (Figure 4.3).

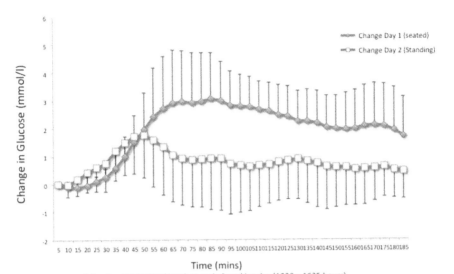

Change in blood glucose, following a standard buffet lunch, whilst working predominantly for 185 mins in a seated or standing position (n=9)

**FIGURE 4.3** Blood glucose levels decline more quickly after lunch when standing than when sitting. (Source: Adapted from Buckley et al. (2014), with permission.)

One possible reason for the difference is that the circulation of blood through the body is greater in standing than in sitting. When sitting, the leg muscles, in particular, are relaxed whereas, when standing, more of the antigravity muscles are active to brace the limbs and maintain balance. In order for glucose to be absorbed from the blood, the blood must reach target tissues that are sensitive to insulin and muscles are a prime target. The large muscle groups in the lower limbs are better perfused when standing and therefore there are more sites available to absorb glucose. Peddie et al. (2013) found that even small movements were sufficient to improve glucose metabolism after eating even if they barely increased heart rate (fidgeting, visiting the bathroom, standing instead of sitting).

Another benefit of swapping sitting for standing after lunch relates to the human body clock. Many physical and psychological processes follow a 24-hour ("circadian") rhythm. After lunch, there is a "post lunch dip" often experienced as drowsiness and lassitude. Standing after lunch improves circulation and may counter these effects.

Given the trend in diabetes since the 1950s, and that those with this condition cannot regulate their blood glucose effectively, moving at work, particularly after lunch may be particularly beneficial. However, in order to achieve the beneficial reductions in blood glucose levels, the volunteers in Buckley's experiments had to stand for three hours after lunch. As we shall see in the next chapter, standing for this length of time brings its own problems which need to be understood in order for better work practices and habits to be introduced successfully.

## KEY POINTS

1. If sitting for 8 hours per day is a health hazard independently of leisure-time exercise, are we putting our office staff at risk if they can only work in a seated position?

2. Energy expenditure when standing is not much greater than when sitting and substituting sitting for two hours per day with standing is unlikely to result in weight loss in overweight or obese people. Standing more at work may bring other health benefits though.

3. Has office design been "overtaken by events"? Does new evidence on health and sedentary work call for a radical rethink in the way we work and the way offices are designed?

4. Time spent sitting per day and participation in exercise are independent risk factors for the development of health problems. To get the best outcome, most people should sit less and exercise more.

5. Has sedentary work become unhealthy due to demographic change? If it has, what can we do about it?

6. Standing more at work for two hours per day would be unlikely to have any useful effect on reducing body fatness or be useful in the treatment of obesity.

7. Limit sitting time at work to less than four hours per day. Although this guidance is not yet definitive (the advice has not been tested in a prospective study) there is sufficient evidence that together with sitting when commuting and at home, most of us would fall into the "moderate" sedentary group of four to eight hours/day where the health risks are lower (Katzmarzyk et al., 2009).

8. Build movement into sedentary jobs. Do:
   a. Encourage users of sit-stand desks to stand after lunch
   b. Site catering facilities away from the office
   c. Hold meetings at standing desks after lunch
   d. Discourage employees from eating at their desks.

9. While many jobs require employees to sit all day, they are not required to smoke tobacco while doing so and in many offices smoking is banned. In this sense sitting is most definitely **NOT** the new smoking.

# 5 Are We Built to Stand?

## Problems with Standing at Work and How to Avoid Them

There is general agreement that stance is steadied when the eyes are open and focussed on a fixed point, and least stable with the eyes closed. ... Posture is essentially an automatism and the mind is unaware of how we do our standing.

**Sherrington (1933)**

We saw earlier that the concept of "correct" sitting used to design chairs was found to be lacking and many sedentary workers suffered discomfort. We also reviewed some of the evidence that a sedentary lifestyle is harmful, and evidence for the benefits of standing and moving, particularly after lunch

*Is standing really any better and if we are to stand more at the office, what's the best way to stand, what might go wrong and what kind of advice can we give employees who want to stand at their desks?*

Evidence from studies of the introduction of sit-stand workstations indicates that the reduction in sitting time at work is modest. Although estimates vary, most studies show reductions of less than two hours per day, much less than the three hours of standing after lunch that took place in the study of blood glucose levels. One study by Vink et al. (2009) found that over a two-week period working six hours per day, people working at sit-stand desks only stood for about 8 percent of the time.

*What is it about standing that people dislike?*

## ARE WE BUILT TO STAND?

The short answer is "no" – human beings are not built to stand, at least not to *stand still* and not for any length of time. It is unnatural, uncomfortable and unhealthy for the following reasons:

1. Blood pools in the lower legs
2. Pressure on the joints causes discomfort and strain
3. Problems such as varicose veins, hip joint degeneration are higher in occupations where people have to stand (Bridger, 2018).

Human beings are extremely well adapted to *walking* on two legs but not to standing and certainly not to standing still. Melzack (1977) gave an extreme example that well-illustrates this fact. Miss C was a young Canadian with a condition known as "congenital insensitivity to pain" – she had never felt pain. Even when she was exposed to painful stimuli such as heat or extreme cold, she felt no pain and there were none of the physiological responses that normally occur when people feel pain (increases in heart rate, blood pressure and so on). Sadly, she developed serious hip, knee and spine problems and died of infections to these joints. Her surgeon attributed these problems to the lack of protection normally provided to the joints by shifting your body weight, fidgeting, changing posture and noticing uncomfortable postures. These behaviors prevent inflammation of the joints and are prompted by feelings of discomfort.

The moral of the story is that standing still or adopting any other kind of fixed posture for any length of time is unhealthy and the best way to avoid discomfort is to avoid fixed postures. In this chapter and the next few chapters, we will look at some of the ways to do this in the office.

It has been known for a very long time that the circulation of blood in the lower extremities when standing still is greater than that in other parts of the body (Thompson et al., 1928). Prolonged standing in one place is a common cause of leg complaints, varicose veins and other circulatory problems in many occupations such as saleswomen (Grandjean, 1980). Leg complaints are common among industrial workers who have to stand all day. In fact, there are guidelines that limit the amount of time people should stand still at work to avoid discomfort (Dul et al., 1993). When standing still with the feet together, looking straight ahead and with the hands at a height of about three quarters of shoulder height (about the height of a keyboard at a standing desk) the maximum time allowed is just under eight minutes if the hands are close to the body (within about 40cm) and just under four minutes if the hands are held about one half of the maximum forward reach. In general the risk of developing health complaints is greater in static postures (see Figure 1.13).

The aim of this guideline is to prevent discomfort, so, given how uncomfortable it soon becomes when standing still, it is not surprising that office workers will be reluctant to stand still and is one of the reasons why sedentary work became the norm in offices over 100 years ago.

## PEOPLE NEVER STAND STILL UNLESS THEY HAVE TO

As we saw in Chapter 1, in everyday life, people almost never stand still, with both feet together, looking straight ahead, except, perhaps, when waiting to cross the road and "standing to attention." Standing this way is really only a transitional or ceremonial posture that people rarely adopt spontaneously. Typically, people stand with the weight predominantly on one foot and often with the right foot forward and the toes pointing slightly to the right. This improves balance by making the base of support at the feet larger and enables the muscles in one leg to rest. Alternating between legs helps to prevent foot swelling, as is explained below.

## POSTURAL SWAY WHEN STANDING
## TO WORK AT A COMPUTER

A study by Foster et al. (1998) had subjects in a laboratory carry out a computerized memory task while standing (Figure 5.1). Postural sway was measured and compared with the amount of sway occurring when the subjects were asked to stand as still as they could. There was *barely any difference in sway*, indicating that standing to work at a computer is no different from standing still when one is absorbed in a task. In fact, working at a computer terminal is almost guaranteed to immobilize a standing worker because the eyes are focussed on a fixed point (the screen) and the hands are working on the keyboard or mouse.

Furthermore, we are unaware of how immobile we really are – at least until discomfort sets in and we have the urge to sit down!

The technical word for this kind of immobilization caused by standing to work at a computer is *"postural fixity."* Like poor old Pope Gregory in Chapter 2, the standing computer worker has few options for changing position while working unless we design the workplace and the job to encourage more movement.

Postural fixity – when standing still – brings its own problems, as is described below.

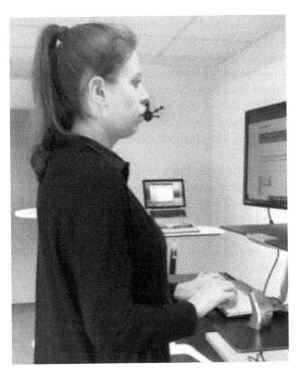

**FIGURE 5.1**   It has been known since the 1930s that when people stand still and focus on a fixed target, they stand *very still*. When standing to carry out intensive screen-based work, people will stand still – as a result, discomfort, mainly in the legs, will be experienced in around 20 minutes. (Source: Foster et al., 1998.)

## PROBLEMS OF STANDING STILL

The heart pumps blood to the lower limbs through the arteries, assisted by gravity. The return of blood to the heart via the veins is opposed by gravity. Standing still causes blood to pool in the lower limbs due to the effects of gravity. Cardiac output is reduced when standing compared to lying down because of the pooling of blood in the lower limbs – there is less blood returning to the heart and therefore less blood available to carry oxygen to other parts of the body.

Plasma in the circulating blood is reduced when standing still after about 20–30 minutes and is restored in about the same time when reclining (Sherrington, 1933). There is a progressive increase in leg and foot volume when standing still and, in general, circulation of the blood is less adequate when standing still, which is why people are more likely to faint when standing still than when walking or sitting down.

In extreme cases, some people may experience *"orthostatic hypotension"* (a sudden drop in blood pressure) when moving from a seated to a standing position. The symptoms are dizziness or light-headedness when standing up which occurs as a result of abnormal blood pressure regulation. Normally, when people stand, gravity causes blood to pool in the veins of the legs and trunk. This pooling lowers the blood pressure and the amount of blood available for the heart to pump to the brain. People with low blood pressure (90/60mmHg or lower) may be more likely to experience these symptoms when standing up and the symptoms normally subside in 10 minutes. In extreme cases, "fainters" may be at risk within 10 to 30 minutes of standing.

Orthostatic hypotension is related to standing still It is characterized by a chief complaint of marked weakness on standing, blurred vision, dizziness and fainting. Lowering the head, sitting or lying down bring complete relief. Warm weather makes things worse because blood is circulated to the skin to cool the body, leaving even less blood available to be pumped to the brain. Dehydration and anemia also increase the risk of fainting.

Pooling of blood in the lower limbs is reduced when we walk or move our feet because contraction of the muscles in the legs, particularly the lower legs, squeezes the veins and forces blood back to the heart. This has benefits for maintaining a steady heart rate and preventing any feeling of dizziness. *The calf muscles play a major role in returning blood to the heart when we stand or walk which explains why it is important when standing to work at a computer that movement of the feet is unrestrained.* There should be plenty of free space under desks to allow standing computer users to move their feet. As we shall see below, there are good reasons for installing footrests for workers to use when standing.

## EVERY LITTLE HELPS

The calf muscles are one of the main antigravity muscles that enable us to stand upright (they prevent the body from jackknifing forwards over the ankle joints). Even though the activity of these muscles is low when we stand quietly, light activity of all these large muscles in the lower limbs may well supply sufficient compression to move a significant quantity of blood back to the heart. Without movement, adequate return of blood to the heart is difficult to maintain even in healthy people when the vertical stance must be sustained for protracted periods of time. Postural sway is also important. Hellebrandt and Franseen (1943) found that only when postural sway was *unrestrained*, could people tolerate standing still for one hour.

The main problem with standing still to do office work is that we can't do most of the things that people naturally do when standing – as described in Chapter 1. Standing to work at a computer for any length of time will inevitably lead to discomfort and possibly foot swelling.

## FOOT SWELLING

Swelling of the feet occurs both when sitting, when standing at work and on long flights. There is a 66 percent reduction in blood flow in the veins of the lower leg during long periods of inactive sitting. Leg volume can increase by 5 percent over a working day.

*For both seated and standing workers, lack of leg movement is a major cause of foot swelling.*

Plantar flexion of the ankle joint (pointing the toes downwards when sitting, or standing on tip-toe) activates the muscle pump (mainly through contraction of the soleus, or calf muscles) and pumps blood back up to the heart against gravity.

Several researchers have investigated foot swelling in prolonged standing. Rys and Konz (1994) found a small (less than 1 percent) difference in foot volume when standing for 240 minutes compared to sitting – in other words, foot swelling when standing was very similar to sitting. The mean foot volume increase was 1.4 percent during the experiment and the footprint area of the feet was 6.7 percent larger at 240 minutes than at the beginning. The width of the instep area at its narrowest point increased 8.6 percent and, at its maximum point, it increased by 3 percent. The foot length did not change over time, indicating that most of the swelling takes place in the midfoot. This means that blood pooling takes place in the feet and, combined with lowering the arches, the width of the foot increases.

Foot swelling occurs more rapidly in the mornings than in the afternoon in both sedentary daytime employees and in those who stand (Belczak et al., 2009). This is because the limbs in the early morning are free from edema (build-up of bodily fluids) because the fluid that accumulated during the previous day has drained from the legs during sleep. On rising to go to work, the legs, now in the upright position, are submitted to gravitational forces. They are akin to a "dry sponge" that fills up quickly within the first few hours if the leg muscles are inactive. The edema that occurs during the morning may reduce the speed of swelling during the afternoon as the pressure in the limbs builds up. This implies that to reduce the discomfort and feelings of fatigue due to leg swelling, employees should maintain a level of physical activity that stimulates the leg muscle throughout the day. Examples include, standing on "tip-toe," walking for 2 minutes every 15 minutes, walking up and down the stairs or using a foot pump device (Figure 5.2).

In general, standing workers should not have to stand on hard concrete floors. This soon leads to discomfort and more rapid swelling of the feet. Instead, many industries use so-called "anti-fatigue mats" to prevent discomfort in employees who

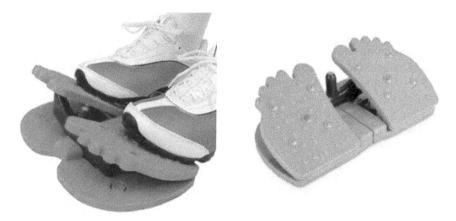

**FIGURE 5.2**  Example of a device designed to encourage foot movement and activation of the venous pump when sitting (Sitting Stepper Available at StressNoMore.co.uk.)

have to stand all day. These mats are suitable for office workers who wish to stand, particularly if the floors have concrete or unyielding surfaces (Figure 5.3).

Prolonged standing causes significant localized leg muscle fatigue, particularly in the calf muscles (one of the main antigravity muscles described earlier in the chapter that is essential for the operation of the "ankle strategy").

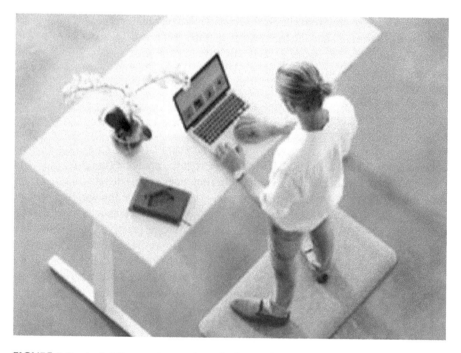

**FIGURE 5.3**  Anti-fatigue mats to reduce tiredness when standing on hard floors. (Source: photo courtesy of Office Reality Ltd., Officereality.co.uk.)

Paul (1995) conducted a controlled field study of the effect of sit-stand workstations on foot swelling during the course of a workday in visual display terminal (VDT) operators. Six VDT operators first worked in offices furnished with nonadjustable sitting workstations. Then they worked in offices furnished with sit-stand adjustable furniture for six weeks. In the later setting, they stood for 15 minutes every hour. In both settings, the foot swelling was measured at 8 a.m., 12 p.m., 1 p.m. and 5 p.m. using a foot volumeter. Between 12 p.m. and 1 p.m., subjects walked for 20 minutes and sat for 40 minutes. The results showed that the average right foot swelling in offices with sit-stand adjustable furniture was significantly less than that in offices with nonadjustable furniture, 12.3 ml (1.1 percent) compared to 21 ml (1.8 percent). These results suggest that the activity promoted using sit-stand workstations benefits sedentary office workers.

For employees already suffering from chronic venous insufficiency and who wish to increase the time they spend standing at work, compression stockings may be beneficial in preventing foot swelling (Krijnen et al., 1997).

## VARICOSE VEINS AND CHRONIC VENOUS INSUFFICIENCY: ARE 21ST CENTURY WORKERS FIT TO STAND?

*Chronic venous insufficiency* is a condition in which the walls and/or the valves in the leg veins are not working properly. In the long term, it can cause serious problems such as bleeding or deep vein thrombosis.

Varicose veins are veins in which the valves function ineffectively. Veins have one-way valves in them so that when the leg muscles contract, the veins are squeezed and blood moves up the vein towards the heart. The valves stop the blood from flowing back when the muscles relax. In people with varicose veins, fluid accumulates in the lower limbs more rapidly because the valves don't work properly. This is why the action of the antigravity muscles is so important for proper circulation when we are standing still. When the problem occurs in deep veins, the blood may return along abnormal pathways and lead to long-term health problems such as chronic edema (chronically swollen legs caused by the pooling of body fluids) and leg ulcers.

As was discussed in the previous chapter, demographic changes have occurred in the last 50 years, resulting in a larger percentage of the population being overweight or obese and lacking exercise. These factors increase the risk of vascular problems such as varicose veins. Other risk factors include the aging of the workforce, a family history of venous disease, pregnancy and *working in an occupation where employees have to stand still*.

These risk factors, together with high blood pressure and cigarette smoking increase the likelihood of chronic venous insufficiency. The disease is one of the ten leading causes of hospitalization in Denmark (Tomei et al., 1999). Epidemiological studies have suggested that up to 15 percent of men and 25 percent of women in the United Kingdom have visible varicose veins (Bradbury et al., 1999) and more than 50,000 varicose vein operations are performed each year in England and Wales. The direct annual cost to the UK's National Health Service of treating chronic venous insufficiency is estimated at £400–600m.

Tuchsen (2000) followed 1.6 million Danish workers for three years from 1991. Men who worked mostly in a standing position were almost twice as likely to be hospitalized for varicose veins compared to all others. Women who worked standing were 2.5 times more likely to be hospitalized. A study by Tomei et al. (1999) reported the findings of an investigation of chronic venous diseases (major and minor) in office workers, industrial workers and stoneworkers. The prevalence of disorders was higher among industrial workers (39.28 percent) than among stoneworkers (24.16 percent, P=.019) and office workers (22.11 percent, P=.010). Within these groups, those employees who spent more than 50 percent of their shift standing were at higher risk of developing the disease.

Given these findings, we might question whether it is desirable to encourage office workers to stand at their desks? Clearly there are arguments for and against. *In the section below, we will review evidence-based guidance for standing to work to minimize the risks.*

## FLOOR MATS AND CARPETS ARE BETTER THAN HARD, COLD FLOORS

There are many reasons why employees should not have to stand on cold, hard floors. Carpets or resilient rubber floor mats (or similar) are often used to provide a more yielding surface and there is evidence that they are effective in reducing fatigue and foot swelling. An experiment by Rys and Konz (1989) showed that, after 60 minutes of standing on mats, as opposed to hard concrete floors, footprint area increased about 1.5 percent less than when their subjects stood on concrete. Footprint area is a measure of foot swelling (to measure footprint area, people stand on a surface with talcum powder on a black card. The powder that sticks to the feet gives an indication of the contact areas of the foot and the floor; the more the foot swells, the greater the contact area). In another experiment, 20 subjects stood for 120 minutes on both concrete and industrial carpet (Rys and Konz, 1989). The mean heart rate when standing on carpet was 5 percent lower than for concrete and the difference was statistically significant. Heart rate at the end of 120 minutes was 8 percent lower than at the start time. Rys and Konz (1989) had nine subjects stand 60 minutes on two mats and on concrete. Over time, discomfort increased on all parts of the body with the shoulder experiencing the least increase in discomfort (24 percent) and the heel the most (57 percent). One mat was more comfortable (than concrete) for upper back, mid back and low back but both mats were more comfortable than concrete.

## PHYSICAL ACTIVITY LEVELS WHEN STANDING

In the previous chapter, we compared the weekly physical activity levels of a sedentary office worker with a housewife in the 1950s, both working 40 hours per week. Recall that this example was given following a review of the increase in the prevalence of obesity since the 1950s and the evidence that we are not as physically active as we used to be. Using some simplifying assumptions, we found that in order to be as physically active as a 1950s housewife, the office worker would have to exercise more after work – the equivalent of spending ten hours per week in an aerobics class or five hours per week playing squash!

Suppose the office worker now spends four hours per day standing and four hours sitting. What difference will it make to the weekly energy expenditure?

Sedentary screen-based keyboard work has a physical activity level of about 1.45 METS (58 MET hours for a 40-hour week) According to Mansoubi et al. (2015) standing has an activity level of 1.59 METS (a total of 60.8 MET hours for a 40-hour week, with four hours standing and four hours sitting per day). The difference is 2.8 MET hours. Comparing 40 hours of sedentary work with 40 hours of sit-stand working where an equal amount of time is spent sitting and standing, the increase in physical activity is the equivalent of doing about 28 minutes of aerobics or 14 minutes of squash per week.

Given that computer-intensive tasks result in a static standing posture, this calculation suggests that standing to operate a computer is unlikely to bring about meaningful increases in the physical activity level of office workers. However, if we assume that the office worker engages in other standing tasks, such as attending meetings, engaging in more face-to-face conversation with employees rather using email and so on, then the physical activity level might approximate that of a bartender or shop assistant – 2.3 METS.

Assuming a 40-hour working week with four hours per day spent sitting and four hours per day in active standing and walking, the office worker now has a weekly work activity level of 76 MET hours – 16 MET hours more than the sedentary worker. The difference in physical activity levels is equivalent to spending 2.7 hours per week in an aerobics class or 1.33 hours per week playing squash (we'll ignore for the moment that there are likely to be additional benefits of vigorous exercise such as squash and that the extra activity is not exactly equivalent to participating in these sports).

*Standing, on its own, is barely more active than sitting. Physical activity levels can be increased further, by using the stairs instead of the escalators, walking to meetings etc.*

## ONSET OF DISCOMFORT WHEN STANDING STILL

Basmajian (1978) pointed out that, once in the upright posture, humans have the most economical antigravity mechanism of all animals. Fatigue is associated with direct tensions on inert structures and circulatory inadequacies. In other words, although standing still is energy efficient it is not biomechanically efficient due to the constant pressure on the feet, pooling of blood in the legs and so on.

Foster et al. (1998) observed subjects in an experiment who stood at a computer for one hour during which time they carried out a repetitive mental task. No reading off-screen or writing was required and only simple keyboard actions were carried out. Very accurate measurements of postural sway were made and compared to the sway measured when subjects were told to stand still but were not working at the computer. The result was that subjects stood very still. Discomfort, mainly in the legs started to become apparent after 25 minutes and steadily increased up to 45 minutes of standing after which it increased more rapidly (Figure 5.4).

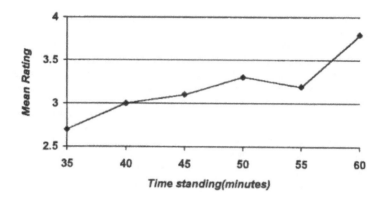

**FIGURE 5.4**    Ratings of discomfort (1 to 5 where a higher score indicates more discomfort) when standing to work at a computer for one hour. Discomfort, mainly in the legs is fairly mild for the first 20–25 minutes before it increases, increasingly rapidly towards the hour.

All of Foster's subjects were healthy, young people with no history of circulatory insufficiency or back problems. It is likely that many older or obese employees would experience discomfort much sooner if asked to perform similar tasks when standing.

## FOOTWEAR FOR STANDING AT WORK

As we have seen already, when people stand for long periods, swelling of the feet takes place in a matter of hours.

Rys and Konz (1990) had nine male subjects in their experiment stand for 240 minutes. Foot volume had increased 1.4 percent by 240 minutes. The minimum width of the instep area had increased by 8.690 percent while the maximum width of the instep had increased only 3 percent. Foot length did not change. *This suggests that most of the swelling takes place in the midfoot.*

Rhys and Konz recommend that shoes that have laces at the ball and top are the best choice as this type of shoe will allow for expansion to take place. They also recommended that when shoes are used for standing work they should be ½ to 1 size larger than normal to allow for the fact that the feet will swell. When buying shoes for standing work, users should buy them after work when their feet are already swollen (not at the weekend).

How do people who have to stand still cope? Guards at the UK's royal palaces have to stand still for long periods. Konz and Johnson (2007) quote a Buckingham Palace guard as follows, "*Stood on parade for four or five hours at a time. The trick is to keep the weight off your heels. That's why guards' boots bulge out in front – plenty of room to wiggle your toes.*"

## HIGH-HEELED SHOES

Should standing workers wear high-heeled shoes? Reports of discomfort in the feet, front of the legs and lower back are likely to be due to the effect wearing such shoes has on the loading of the feet and legs and on standing posture. Speksnijder et al. (2005)

compared women wearing high-heeled (6cm) and flat-heeled (1cm) shoes. Wearing high-heeled shoes increased pressure on the forefoot by 40 percent and the authors suggested that diabetics and those with rheumatoid arthritis should avoid wearing high-heeled shoes at work.

Lee et al. (2001) investigated the mechanical effects of wearing shoes with different heel heights (0, 4.5 and 8cm). When wearing high-heeled shoes, people counteract the tendency to fall forwards by flexing the ankles (leaning back slightly) which places a load on the muscles at the front to the shin and on the muscles in the lower back.

It is sometimes thought that wearing high-heels causes people to arch their backs and that this is the cause of back pain. The evidence suggests that, if anything, the opposite happens, and the lumbar curve is flattened. Together with increased back muscle activity, this will result in increased and abnormal loading of the lower part of the spine which is a cause of discomfort.

*As a general rule, high-heeled shoes are not recommended for office work conducted standing because they increase the pressure on the front part of the foot and cause a slightly unbalanced posture that leads to discomfort over time.*

## FLOOR SPACE

Why is space for the feet so important? Floor space is important so that users can stand close to the front of the desk to access the keyboard and work documents. In a study by Whistance et al. (1995), subjects stood at a computer to work for one hour and different workstation arrangements were compared. In one condition, a board was placed below the front of the desk to constrain the position of the feet. With the constrained foot position, the front of the subject's foot could not go under the bench, forcing the subject to stand further back and to compensate by increased flexion at the hips. The constrained foot position also resulted in increased plantar flexion (leaning backwards from the ankles). This could be accounted for by subjects placing their feet as far forward as they could go while increased forward flexion at the hips resulted in compensatory backwards displacement of the ankles. The net effect of these changes was to increase the static muscle load on the back and the risk of back pain.

## FOOTRESTS FOR STANDING WORKERS?

Footrests have long been recommended for seated work with computers because they help stabilize the sitter and reduce pressure under the thighs, providing a greater variety of foot positions – what about standing workers?

We saw in Chapter 1 that the human body is well designed for walking and this requires standing on one leg for part of the time (as the other leg swings through for the next step). In fact, the ability to maintain postural stability when standing on one leg is one of the reasons why human beings can walk upright on two legs far more efficiently than any other primates.

The ability to do this is due to the shape of the pelvis. The human pelvis is very different from that of modern chimpanzees and gorillas (Figure 5.5).

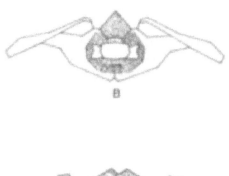

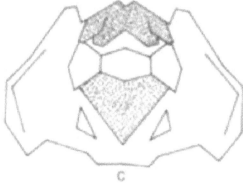

FIGURE 5.5   Comparison of the human and chimpanzee pelvic bones ("ilia"). Seen from above, the chimpanzee has a flat pelvis (upper figure), whereas in the human pelvis the iliac bones are curved to the sides to stabilize the pelvis laterally when we walk.

Seen from above the bones of the human pelvis curve to the side. When you put your hands in your pockets, you can feel your pelvic bones. These are known as the iliac bones and they are on either side of the body at the level of the waist (in fact, waistbands and belts rest on the top of the iliac bones, in a region known as the "iliac crest"). In other primates these bones do not curve to the side, they are flat (Figure 5.5).

In humans, a group of muscles known as the "anterior gluteals" attach the side of the thigh bone (the femur) to the pelvis at the side of the body, on the curved part of the iliac bone, approximately at the level of one's trouser pockets. When we walk with the weight supported on one leg as the other leg swings through, the anterior gluteal muscles on the side supporting the body weight contract to stop the pelvis tilting towards the unsupported side of the body. This is why we don't sway from side to side when we walk.

You can demonstrate this easily by placing your fingertips firmly over the iliac bones on both sides of your body at about the level of your trouser pockets. Stand still with your weight balanced equally on both feet. The anterior gluteal muscles will feel soft. Now walk forwards – your will feel the muscles contract and relax as you walk. As one leg swings through the muscles on that side relax and the muscles on the other side contract in time with the swinging leg (Figure 5.6).

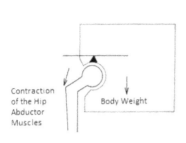
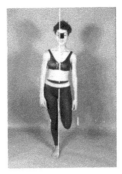
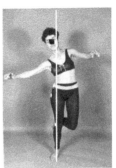

Contraction
of the Hip
Abductor
Muscles

Body Weight

**FIGURE 5.6** Humans are well adapted to standing on one leg due to the curved shape of the pelvis and the hip abductor muscles. When we walk, these muscles contract to stop us falling to the side. If these muscles fail, the upper body has to compensate to maintain balance.

In other primates the pelvis is flat and all the gluteal muscles work together to extend the hip – to push the animal forwards when walking. That is one of the reasons why, when chimpanzees and gorillas do walk upright, they tend to sway from side to side – the upper body has to sway over the supporting leg to maintain balance and stop the animal falling to the unsupported side.

Interestingly, the curve in the iliac bones of the pelvis was a major evolutionary step that enabled our hominin ancestors to develop energy efficient walking. Like the lumbar curve ("lumbar lordosis") described in Chapter 1, the adaptation of the pelvis enables us to walk without having to compensate for standing on one leg by moving the upper body to the side to maintain balance. Modern human beings are not the only ones to have had this remodeling of the pelvis. It seems that all our hominin ancestors, going back to Australopithecus Afarensis which roamed the plains of Africa 4 million years ago, were all well adapted to walking upright in an energy efficient way (Lovejoy, 1988). The downside of the evolutionary remodeling of the pelvis was that the space for giving birth to offspring was reduced at a time in evolutionary history when the size of hominin brains was increasing!

## STANDING ON ONE LEG IS NORMAL

In daily life, people normally stand with the body weight mainly on one leg, shifting to the other from time to time. This provides a natural cycle of work and rest for the legs – almost like walking on the spot in slow motion. It activates the venous pump.

Footrests provide a similar function – even today, suppliers of furniture and fittings for pubs and bars sell footrails to enable their customers to stand more comfortably at the bar (Figure 5.7). The crime author, Ian Rankin, described how his detective character,

> … would prop up the Oxford Bar in Edinburgh "with an IPA in his hand and his feet resting on the rail."

Anecdotally, there is an Oxford Bar in Edinburgh but it didn't have a footrail installed. When the landlord heard the story, he had one installed!

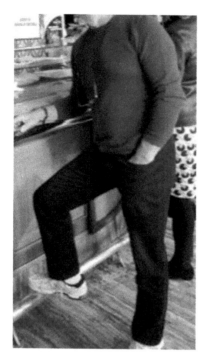

**FIGURE 5.7** Footrails for comfortable standing are less common than they used to be despite the natural tendency of people to use objects around them for support. They can still be found in Public Houses in many parts of the world.

Placing one foot on a footrest does more than rest the leg. It changes the posture of the body because the hip on the footrest side is flexed slightly. Bridger and Orkin (1992) measured the effect of a footrest on standing posture. They found that a footrest that raised the resting foot 250mm above the floor caused the pelvis on the same side of the body to tilt backwards by about 4–6 degrees (Figure 5.8), relaxing the iliopsoas and back muscles on that side and improving blood flow. The supporting leg was straightened and the ankle plantar-flexed (as the weight of the body moved back over the heels).

Satzler et al. (1993) did a study of footrests using four conditions: (1) standing with one foot on a 100mm flat platform; (2) standing with one foot on a 100mm, 15-degree angled platform; (3) standing with one foot on a 100mm high 50mm diameter bar; and (4) (control) standing with both feet flat on a concrete floor. Sixteen subjects stood for two hours in each of the four conditions. The subjects were videotaped while standing and were permitted to shift their feet between the floor and the footrest at will. The three footrests were preferred over no footrest (control); of the footrests, the two platforms seemed better than the bar. The percentage of time a foot was on the footrest was 59 percent for the bar, 75 percent for the inclined platform and 83 percent for the flat platform; the 75 percent and 83 percent were not significantly different from each other but both were significantly different from the 59 percent. Subjects switched their foot from the floor to an aid 0.6 times/min

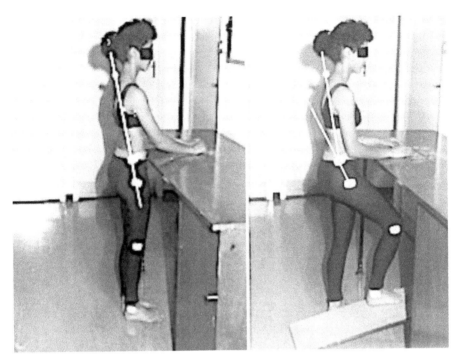

**FIGURE 5.8** Experimental evidence suggests that when standing workers are offered footrests they use them. Apart from activating the venous muscle pump, they cause the pelvis to tip back slightly which some back pain sufferers may find beneficial.

(a switch every 90 seconds) – effectively for 83 percent of the time they used the footrest.

*This is interesting because in comfortable walking about 80 percent of the cycle is spent with the body supported by a single leg. From this point of view, comfortable standing with a footrest is like walking on the spot in slow motion!*

Son et al. (2017) investigated the effects of a foot platform on back muscle activity, discomfort and posture on subjects performing standing computer work for two hours and either standing on a flat surface or using footrests of 5, 10 and 15 percent of their body height.

The lumbar lordosis was less when using all the footrests compared to standing on the flat surface, the activity of the lower back muscles (lumbar erectors spinae) was reduced and the muscles were less fatigued. *Use of a footrest at 10 percent of stature led to the lowest stress on the lumbar region of the back and was recommended as the best option.*

The use of a footrest (Figure 5.9) seems to be a valid way of solving the problem of "postural fixity" when standing to work with computers and laptops and might help prevent back pain in people with symptomatic facet joints (because it flattens the lumbar spine slightly).

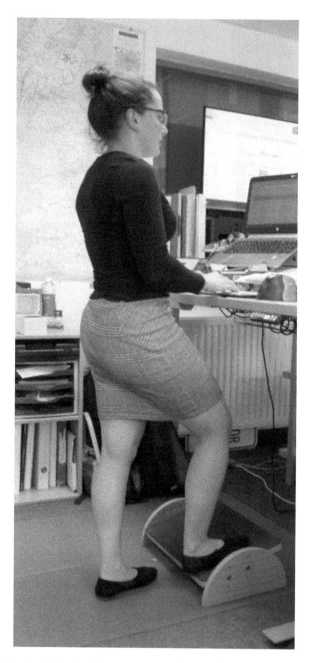

**FIGURE 5.9** Footrests for standing computer work – standing on one leg or walking on the spot in slow motion?

## STATIC POSTURES AND STANDING WORK

We saw in Chapter 1, that static postures and highly repetitive postures increase the risk of health problems and discomfort. In fact, there is an International Standard that gives time limits for static work – ISO 11226 (Delleman and Dul, 2007).

ISO 11226:2000 "Ergonomics – Evaluation of static working postures," which was ratified in 2018, gives time limits for forward inclinations of the trunk when working. These are the maximum times that employees can be expected to maintain a static work position safely:

- Bending forwards by 60 degrees or more is not permitted at all
- Standing leaning backwards to work is not permitted without back support
- Leaning forwards up to 20 degrees is permitted for five minutes maximum
- Leaning forwards 20–60 degrees is permitted for one to four minutes (about two minutes at 45 degrees).

Most office workers who choose to stand to work at their desks are unlikely to lean forwards by more than a few degrees, except if the workstation is adjusted incorrectly.

In Figure 1.6, we can see an employee working at a computer that is too low resulting in the need to tilt the upper body forward.

According to ISO 11226, this posture would be permitted for about five minutes. Quite subtle postural deviations can result in the onset of discomfort and may be one reason why, as we shall see in the following chapters, employees given sit-stand workstations typically do not stand for very long each day.

## BACK PAIN WHEN STANDING

We saw in Chapter 1 that there is no such thing as a "good" posture and people naturally vary their postures throughout the day.

Not everyone experiences backache and there is no single cause of backache. Some people with symptomatic discs in the lower back are more likely to get back pain when they sit down and if they have to bend forwards as when working slumped over a desk (flexing the upper body, like Pope Gregory in Chapter 2) or when bending while working in the garden. Those with degeneration of the facet joints at the back of the spine are more likely to get back pain when standing, because the lower part of the spine is more extended and the load on these joints is greater.

It has been known for many years that back pain is less prevalent in people who sit and stand throughout the day than in people who either sit or stand all day (Magora, 1972) because they are not exposed to potentially uncomfortable postures all day. It seems reasonable to suppose that replacing seated workstations with sit-stand workstations would lower the prevalence of back pain.

Is this true?

Agarwal et el. (2018) reviewed 12 studies of sit-stand workstations and low back pain finding a small reduction in low back discomfort when sit-stand workstations were used. The studies were not able to determine the long-term effects of using the workstations or any long-term implications for the development of chronic problems. Nor were they able to suggest an optimal combination of sitting and standing.

One reason may be that these kinds of interventions are difficult to evaluate in practice due to the so-called "Buffer Effect" (Bendix and Bridger, 2004). The buffer effect is really a kind of compensation for the effects of workstation improvements – people "consume" the increased comfort by working in a given position for a longer period of time. It is the discomfort itself that causes people to change posture, therefore the discomfort doesn't change much even though the workstation is improved.

Given that most back problems are not caused by work (Hartvigsen et al., 2000) these findings are more impressive than they appear at first glance and suggest that sit-stand working is perceived as more comfortable than seated work in those who use it.

Do people actually use their sit-stand workstations and do they use them enough to, make a difference? If they don't, maybe it's because, unlike the typists who worked for the U.S. Navy in 1944, they haven't been trained how to adjust sit-stand workstations properly. Some basic advice is given below.

## WORKSTATION ADJUSTMENT

The more adjustable a workstation the more likely it will be adjusted incorrectly. For sit-stand workstations the following guidelines can be given:
For sitting:

1. Adjust the height of the seat so that the feet are resting firmly on the floor, or on a footrest.
2. The height of the seat should be about 3cm lower than the underside of the thigh and there should be no pressure under the thighs.
3. Check that the front edge of the seat does not dig into the back of the knees when using the backrest or lumbar support. If it does, a shorter seat (from front to back) is needed, like the 1940s typist chair in Chapter 2.
4. Adjust the desk height so that the mid row of keys on the keyboard is at the height of your elbows.
5. Check that the elbow rests on the chair (if provided) do not impinge the front of the desk, forcing you to sit further away from the desk.
6. Check that the underneath of the desk does not compress the upper part of your thighs.
7. Check that the screen is a comfortable distance from your eyes (approximately 70cm although it will depend on your eyesight and preferences for sizing the text: most modern programs have "view" function to vary the font size on the display).
8. Check that the top of the screen is no higher than your eyes when you are sitting comfortably. Use a document holder if you have to direct your gaze to the screen and to documents during the task.

For Standing:

1. Stand in an upright, comfortable position and look straight ahead.
2. Adjust the desk height so that the mid row of keys on the keyboard is at the height of your elbows.

3. For electrically adjustable/automatic desks, standing elbow height is about 63 percent of stature. So a female 1.65m tall would need a desk height of about 1.04 m. A male 1.80m tall would need a desk height of about 1.13m.

4. Ensure that there is space for the feet underneath and all around the desk.

5. Check that the footrest (if provided) is approximately 15cm distant from the front edge of the desk (so that you can stand close to the desk and move one foot forward under the desk and onto the footrest).

6. Check that you can use the footrest with either foot.

7. Check that the footrest is approximately 10 percent of your stature with the footwear you are using.

8. Check that the screen is still a comfortable viewing distance from your eyes when you transition from sitting to standing. When people sit at a desk they often sit about 15–20cm from the front of the desk, resting their wrists on the desktop or on a wrist rest). When they stand to work, they stand they often move closer to the desk, reducing the distance between the eyes and the screen (Figure 5.10). You may need to move the screen further back when you stand to work.

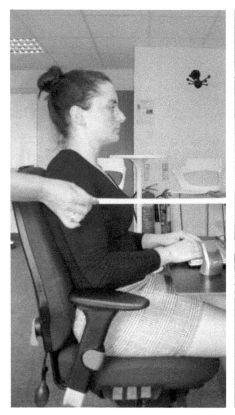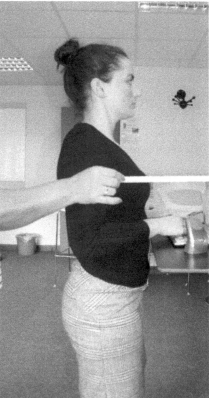

**FIGURE 5.10** Transitioning from sitting to standing. When sitting, people normally recline. When they stand up the upper body is more upright and the eyes closer to the screen.

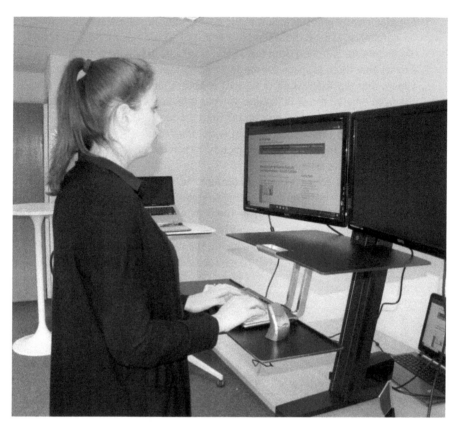

**FIGURE 5.11** Height adjustable platform with inclined pillar – as the screen is raised it moves away from the front of the desk. (Source: Workfit-S by ERGOTRON®, ergotron.com.)

9. Some height-adjustable platforms for sit-stand computer working have an inclined pillar such that the screen moves away from the user as the height is raised, which may compensate for the user moving closer to the desk when standing (Figure 5.11).

## KEY POINTS

1. Standing still at a sit-stand workstation for more than 50 percent of a workday is not recommended if it is conducted over many years.
2. Changing from sitting to standing at sit-stand desks. People often sit about 20cm from the desk when working with a computer. The screen is placed at a comfortable viewing distance. This is not necessarily a comfortable distance when standing close to the desk. Users may stand back and adopt an uncomfortable posture to operate the keyboard.
3. Minimum requirements for foot space. What is the minimum amount of foot space needed under a desk for standing employees? According to Konz and Johnson (2007), "We recommend to keep the numbers simple

and to tell engineers (and designers) to make the space at least 150mm deep, 150mm high and 500mm wide. (In U.S. units, this would be 6 inches deep, 6 inches high, and 20 inches wide.")

4. What makes a floor surface comfortable to stand on? Floor mats are more comfortable to stand on than hard floors because they encourage small postural adjustments that improve circulation in the legs. Rys and Konz (1989) compared the comfort of standing on concrete or three mats of different compressions. A mat with 5.8 percent compression was found to be more comfortable than mats with 7.4 percent and 18.6 percent compression – that is, the firmer mat was more comfortable. Mats should be 1–2cm thick depending on the surface on which they are placed.

5. Mats also provide better friction, aid postural stability and provide better insulation if the floor is cold.

6. Maximum recommended time for static standing – one hour when standing at a computer or doing any kind of work where a static position must be maintained (although 20 minutes at a time is more realistic). Static postures are more likely when doing intensive work at a computer with the eyes focussed mainly on the screen.

7. What kinds of office work are best done standing? The evidence reviewed in the chapter indicates that the best kinds of office work to do at a standing desk are those that require or permit movement and do not require that that the eyes have to be focussed at a fixed point or target, such as a computer screen, for example:
   a. Speaking on the phone
   b. Attending a meeting at a standing table
   c. Reading a hand-held document or book
   d. Any task that requires handling light loads (e.g., sorting papers or reports) is better done standing than sitting because the load on the spine is lower in standing to begin with.

8. What kinds of office work are best done sitting? Intensive computer work, such as programming: data entry; proofreading etc.

9. Users of sit-stand workstations can increase their physical activity levels by engaging in "active standing" – making more use of face-to-face meetings with colleagues instead of email, not eating at their desks and so on. However, since the physical activity levels of sedentary computer work and standing computer work are little different, sedentary employees would benefit in the same way.

10. It is unlikely that employees will stand still at their desks for longer than about 20 minutes or half an hour. Consider using high desks or a table for standing as the norm and providing stools so that standing workers can alternate between standing and sitting without having to adjust the height of the desk.

11. When buying shoes to wear at work at a sit-stand workstation, buy them at the end of the day, when you have been standing to allow for foot swelling. Try shoes ½ to 1 size larger than normal.

12. Freedom to stand with one foot forwards and elevated is an important feature of a well-designed workspace. The evidence suggests that when workstations for standing workers are fitted with footrests, people do use them – for up to 80 percent of the time they spend standing, alternating each foot after short periods of rest.

13. What does a good footrest look like? Platforms are preferred to rails and should be usable by both feet. A foot rest for standing workers should be about 10 percent of stature. A sloping platform (15 degrees) 1500–2000mm should fit most workers. The evidence supports the well-established, and not to be forgotten, view of orthopedic experts that raising one foot onto a rail or footrest will result in a standing posture that is stable while leaving the hands free and, most importantly, is deemed to prevent excessive spinal curvatures and thus remove stress from the intravertebral discs (White and Panjabi, 1990; Fahrni, 1966).

14. ISO 11226 gives time limits for the adoption of static postures at work. Working with the trunk inclined over the desk (e.g., standing leaning forwards slightly to look at a low screen) is only permitted for short periods (see main text). Standing workstations that are adjusted in such a way to violate the standard may be a source of discomfort that discourages their use.

15. The evidence to date indicates that sit-stand workstations may benefit sedentary office workers who suffer back pain when sitting at work. Requests by back pain sufferers for sit-stand workstations are supported by the scientific evidence at the time of writing.

# 6 Standing as a Solution

## *Benefits of Becoming More Active at Work*

In biological terms, posture is constant, continuous adaptation.... Standing is in reality movement upon a stationary base ... From this point of view, normal standing on both legs is almost effortless.

**F.A. Hellebrandt (1938)**

It has been known for a long time that exercise is important for maintaining health and a healthy body composition. Figure 6.1 depicts a model of risks to health based on body mass index (BMI) and waist circumference. A BMI greater than 25 is classified as "overweight" and greater than 30 as "obese."

The BMI of individuals is calculated by dividing their body mass in kilograms by their height squared in meters. For example, a man weighing 80kg standing 1.8m tall would have a BMI of 24.7 (80/(1.8x.18)). The model includes waist circumference to account for the fact that very muscular individuals may have a high BMI but be

| BMI | | Waist circumference (cm) | | |
| --- | --- | --- | --- | --- |
| | | Men < 94 | Men 94-101.9 | Men ≥ 102 |
| | | Women <80 | Women 80-87.9 | Women ≥ 88 |
| Underweight | < 18.5 | Should be informed of risk of underweight, refer to unit MO | | |
| Healthy weight | 18.5-24.9 | None | None | Increased |
| Overweight | 25.0-29.9 | None | Increased | High |
| Obese Class I | 30.0-34.9 | Increased | High | Very High |
| Obese Class II | 35.0-39.9 | High | Very High | Extreme |
| Obese Class III | ≥40 | Very High | Extreme | Extreme |

**FIGURE 6.1** Health risk in relation to body mass index and waist circumference.

perfectly healthy. The health risk is associated with high levels of fat, particularly in the abdomen, rather than overall body mass.

## EXERCISE AND BODY MASS INDEX IN THE LONG TERM

Being overweight or obese is related to diet and to physical activity levels. Bridger et al. (2013) reported data on over 1000 individuals followed between 2007 and 2011. People who reported exercising and having physically demanding jobs in 2007 were less likely to be in the high risk categories in 2011. Those reporting exercising daily had waist circumferences about 4cm less, on average, than those who reported that they never did any exercise (Figure 6.2). These findings suggest that one of the benefits of exercise is that it enables the body to use fats in the diet as a source of energy, rather than storing them in the abdomen and at other sites. Of course, alternative explanations are possible – it may be that the people who exercised in this study also ate lower calorie diets over the five-year period, but with large numbers of people in the study, this explanation seems less likely.

Those with a higher BMI in 2007 were more likely to become obese or overweight in 2011, have high blood pressure and report back pain or musculoskeletal disorders five years later. Increases in BMI over the period (putting on weight) were associated with lower subjective health at the end of the study, as was lack of exercise, as reported in 2007.

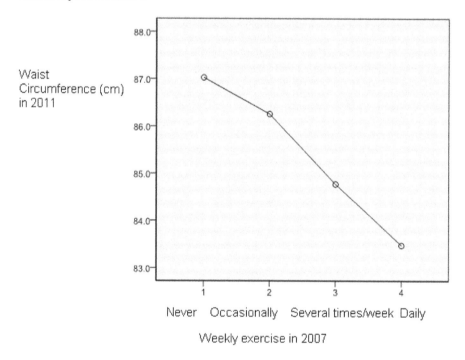

**FIGURE 6.2** Relation between participation in exercise and waist circumference five years later. (Source: from Bridger et al. (2011). Unpublished MOD report, Crown Copyright, contains public sector information licensed under the Open Government Agreement v2.0.)

It is not surprising that heavier people reported more back pain – as we saw earlier, the heaviest weight most of us will ever carry is our own body – the heavier we are, the greater the load on our backs!

## SITTING IS BAD FOR YOU

We saw in Chapter 4 that lack of exercise is only one aspect of an inactive lifestyle that is harmful. Although exercise is beneficial, a sedentary lifestyle is harmful in itself even in those who do exercise. Even in people who exercise, regularly sitting less seems to provide additional benefits. One explanation is simply that exercising outside of work (going for a walk, playing golf, jogging etc.) reduces the time that might otherwise be spent sitting at home.

## TAKING A BREAK FROM SITTING

We have already seen that the greater the total number of hours spent sitting every day, the greater the health risk. There is also evidence that, in addition to the total time spent sitting, *prolonged sitting* (without taking a break) is also harmful.

Healy et al. (2008) found that independently of the total amount of time people spent sitting and independently of the time they spent in moderate-to-vigorous intensity exercise, taking a break from sitting was beneficially associated with the lower levels of metabolic risk variables. These risk variables included elevated levels of triglycerides and plasma glucose, both of which are sources of energy which, ideally, are either used or stored. Triglycerides are breakdown products of the digestion of fat that have been absorbed into the body. Chronically high levels of triglycerides in the blood may raise the risk of heart disease. High plasma glucose levels, as we saw earlier, can damage the walls of blood vessels.

Dunstan et al. (2012) compared the effects of taking a break from sitting every 20 minutes (two-minute breaks of light or moderate walking) with uninterrupted sitting on plasma glucose and insulin levels in overweight and obese volunteers. Interestingly, the total time spent walking over the five hours was negligible in terms of energy expenditure, but was enough to have significant beneficial metabolic effects, providing further evidence that it is the prolonged physical inactivity that is harmful in itself.

Although standing to work at a sit-stand desk is unlikely to cause *weight loss* in overweight people or "burn more calories," taking regular short breaks from sitting is beneficial. Even short breaks of standing while working have been shown to result in increased resistance to fat gain.

## WHY IS PROLONGED SITTING SO HARMFUL?

In Chapter 3, we looked at the bed-rest studies of astronauts to understand why physical inactivity might be harmful. Staying in bed all day was found to cause *"metabolic inflexibility,"* which consisted of a number of unhealthy changes – mainly resistance to the effects of insulin and an inability to control blood sugar levels correctly, together with reduced ability to metabolize fats. The body becomes less able to switch between different energy sources in response to changes in work demands and diet.

It appears that the harmful effects of bed-rest, as observed in NASA's studies of bed-rest in astronauts are essentially the same as those caused by a sedentary lifestyle – effectively metabolic inflexibility (Rynders et al., 2018). The metabolism of healthy people is such that the body can adapt to the kinds of fuel available in the diet (i.e., protein, fats and carbohydrate), to switch between using fat or carbohydrate as the energy source. A sedentary lifestyle reduces the ability to switch between these fuel sources and is a feature of chronic diseases such as Type II diabetes and obesity.

A major cause of metabolic inflexibility seems to be *a lack of skeletal muscle activity*, which is a characteristic of prolonged sedentary behavior (such as sitting looking at screens all day).

*All this evidence suggests that it is not sitting* per se *that is harmful, but the lack of muscle activity that occurs when sitting.*

*So, it might not be necessary to stand more at work in order the gain benefits if employees can become more active even when seated.*

## GETTING PEOPLE TO SIT LESS IN THE OFFICE

Attempts to reduce sitting time at work have had mixed results. Parry et al. (2013) compared three ways of getting office workers to sit less:

*An "Active" Workstation*: Employees had access to treadmill desks and were encouraged to use them for 10 minutes per day building up to 30 minutes per day.

*Inclusion of Traditional Physical Activity*: Promotion of light to moderate activity in breaks between normal office tasks and use of active transport before and after work. Using the stairs instead of the elevator. Employees in this group were given a pedometer for motivation.

*Active Office Ergonomics*: Computer workstation set-up, moving while in the chair (sitting on the front edge), walk and talk meetings

All of the methods brought about reductions in sedentary time at work and in the amount of prolonged sitting. However, the changes were small – less than 2 percent reductions in sedentary time overall and less than one extra break in prolonged sitting per hour. Whether these changes are large enough to have beneficial effects is unknown.

*The evidence to date suggests that merely providing people with the option to stand at work is insufficient to change their behavior.*

## "NUDGING" PEOPLE TO STAND MORE OFTEN

People often have intentions to behave in healthier ways but fail to do so in the face of obstacles, in this case sitting down is easier than overcoming the perceived barriers – standing up from a comfortable chair, raising the desk, adjusting the screen and so on.

Venema et al. (2018) investigated the use of "nudging" techniques to encourage people to stand more when using sit-stand desks. Nudging techniques aim to change behavior by making the desired outcome the "default" option to begin with.

Instead of encouraging sedentary workers to adjust their desks to the standing position throughout the day to reduce sitting time, the researchers adjusted all the desks to the standing position (they were able to do this because employees had no fixed workstations of their own).

Nudging works by relying on the fact that people often take the "path of least resistance" and by setting the desks to standing, people chose to stand rather than adjusting the desk to the sitting position when they arrived at the office.

In the Venema study, some sit-stand desks (SSDs) had been installed in an office three years previously but were hardly ever used to stand at work. The researchers visited the offices regularly and set any empty sitting height desks to standing height. When the employees arrived at work in the morning, the desks were already in the standing position. The researchers also left signs on the desks requesting users to leave the desk at standing height when they had finished working. By changing the default, the researchers introduced slight "friction" – the opposite of nudging – the raised desks were a slight obstacle to working from a seated position, so it was likely that many would choose to stand on arrival at the desk.

Nudging has been successfully applied in a variety of fields and works by making the healthier option the easiest to adopt in circumstances where people have a choice (this may be why organ donor rates are higher in countries where everyone is automatically a donor and non-donors have to "opt-out" compared to countries where donors have to "opt-in").

Prior to the study, the sit-stand desks were seldom used and were adjusted for seated work.

The study showed that "nudging" employees to stand increased the time spent working in a standing position:

- During the baseline measurement 1.82 percent of the employees were working standing up. During the nudge intervention this percentage rose to 13.13 percent.
- Two weeks after the intervention period (i.e., when the SSDs were no longer placed at standing height by default) the stand-up rate was still 10.10 percent. Two months after the nudge intervention the stand-up rate was 7.82 percent.
- There was no evidence that the popularity of the sit-stand workstations changed over the trial period or during follow-up. They were occupied 70–75 percent of the time.
- 56.5 percent of the employees found it acceptable that the workstations were set to standing when they used them (e.g., "I think it is a good idea, I usually just sit down without thinking about it").
- 11.0 percent found it unacceptable (e.g., "I think it is mostly annoying, I don't want to work standing up").
- Finally, 25.4 percent indicated that they had no opinion about it (e.g., "I don't know how long to stand for").
- Most employees had a neutral attitude towards standing to work although there was a social norm that standing was not in favor (drawing attention to oneself or feeling conspicuous).

## PROMPTING PEOPLE TO STAND AT SIT-STAND DESKS

Garrett et al. (2019) investigated the effects of computer-based prompts on users of sit-stand desks. The desks were height adjustable using an electric motor under the user's control and could be pre-set to the required heights for standing and sitting to suit the user. Each user's laptop had software installed that prompted the user to stand for six minutes every half hour. Prompts to stand or sit were delivered by the software but could be postponed by the user for ten minutes. The software monitored the desk height and user's activity throughout the day and the transitions from standing to sitting and vice versa were recorded.

Volunteers in the computer-prompt group were compared over a three-month period with a control group which had the same equipment and software to monitor their behavior, but did not receive any prompts. After three months it was found that the volunteers in the experimental group made more transitions between sitting and standing than those in the control group – in fact, those who were prompted to change from sitting to standing were more than twice as likely to do so. Forty nine percent of the volunteers in the experimental group said they would definitely continue to use the computer prompting software on their laptops and 24 percent said they would probably continue to use it.

The perceived benefits of the behavioral changes prompted by the software were: decreased body discomfort, better mental focus, and improved productivity when combining standing with sitting.

So, computer prompting seems useful in the first few months, at least, in reducing sedentary behavior in the office. Whether it would continue to be effective in the long term is unknown – it may even be unnecessary, as over time, changing posture from sitting to standing might become habitual. Habits, and their development, are a topic that will be returned to in the next chapter.

## PRODUCTIVITY BENEFITS OF SIT-STAND WORKING

Garrett et al. (2016) compared the productivity and self-reported sitting time of call center workers using either traditional sedentary workstations (Figure 6.3) or "stand-capable" workstations where employees could either stand or sit. There were two designs of stand-capable workstations. "Sit-stand" workstations (Figure 6.4) had a traditional office chair that could be adjusted between 40.64cm and 53.34cm. The "stand-biased" workstations (Figure 6.5) had a higher chair that could be adjusted between 64.77cm and 91.44cm together with a foot platform 15–25cm high. Both stand-capable desks had electric height adjustment and could be adjusted at the touch of a button.

Productivity (number of successful call outcomes per hour, where a successful call resulted in revenue) was higher in the stand-capable group by 23 percent in the first month of the study, rising to 53 percent after six months. Employees using stand-capable (both sit-stand and stand-biased) furniture reported sitting for 72–73 percent of the work day compared to 91 percent in those using conventional furniture. Those in the stand-capable group reported less discomfort than those in the sedentary group, which may explain the difference in productivity, which seems to be due to the stand-capable users working more effectively (Figure 6.6),

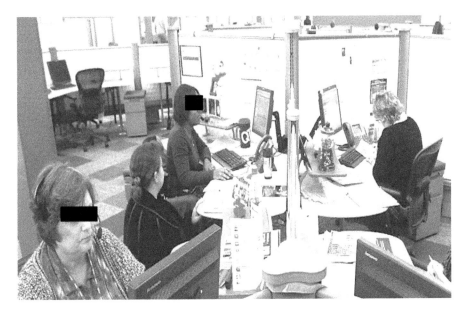

**FIGURE 6.3** Traditional seated workstations in a study of call center productivity. (Source: from: Garrett et al. (2016), with permission.)

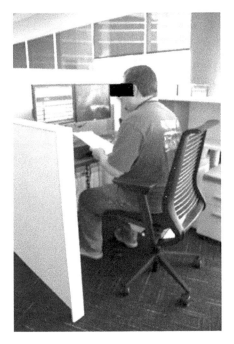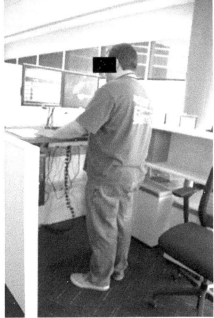

**FIGURE 6.4** Sit-stand workstation in a study of call center productivity. Call center productivity over six months following a standing desk intervention. (Source: Garrett et al. (2016), with permission.)

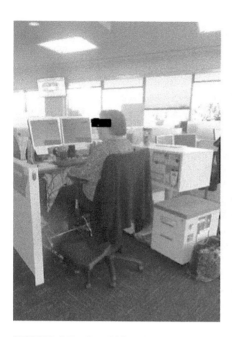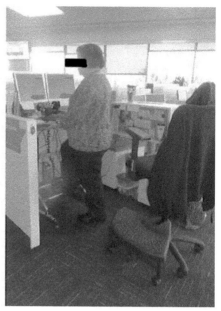

**FIGURE 6.5** Stand-biased workstation – note the use of the footrest when standing and when sitting. Call center productivity over six months following a standing desk intervention. (Source: Garrett et al. (2016), with permission.)

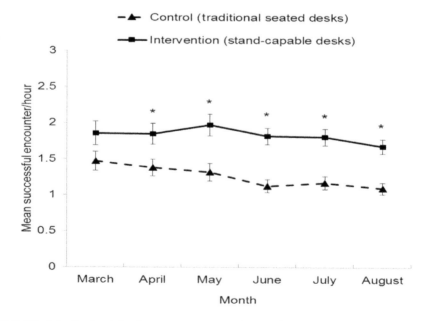

**FIGURE 6.6** Productivity improvements over six months when using sit-stand workstations. Call center productivity over six months following a standing desk intervention. (Source: Garrett et al. (2016), with permission.)

not that they spent more time dealing with calls. The study provides tentative support for productivity enhancement in sit-stand working but the mechanism by which these benefits were achieved is not clear from this study (was it because people are more productive when standing or because there was less distracting discomfort?).

## PRODUCTIVITY AND COMFORT

Karakolis et al. (2016) compared comfort and productivity of 24 volunteers working in a data entry task (typing, reading and data entry). Each volunteer carried out the task in each of three conditions – standing for one hour; sitting for one hour; sit-stand for one hour. The sit-stand condition consisted of 15 minutes sitting followed by 5 minutes standing, repeated over the hour.

The purpose of this study was to investigate the effect of a sit-stand office workstation on standing posture, lower back spine loading, whole back discomfort and task productivity compared to traditional seated and standing workstations.

Volunteers reported less discomfort when working at the sit-stand workstation compared to either sitting or standing, although there was no difference in productivity (possibly because the task was not difficult or because the volunteers didn't spend enough time on the task for productivity differences to appear). Interestingly, volunteers in the sit-stand condition tended to sit up straighter when they did sit down compared to when they only worked in the seated position.

These results provide independent evidence that supports the idea that changing posture prevents the onset of discomfort. The 5:15 ratio for changing from standing to sitting might not be the optimum ratio, but it supports the idea that small, frequent changes are beneficial.

## SIT-STAND WORKSTATIONS, COMFORT AND WORK ABILITY

A study by Ying Gao et al. (2016) investigated time spent sitting in the office as well as the severity of musculoskeletal discomfort ("aches and pains") and work ability in two groups of office workers over a six-month period. One group of 21 volunteers worked at conventional workstations and the other group of 24 volunteers was given sit-stand workstations. The usability of the sit-stand workstations was also assessed using a questionnaire. There was a small but statistically significant reduction in daily sitting time in those with the sit-stand workstations most of which was a replacement of sitting with standing. Users of the sit-stand workstations reported greater musculoskeletal comfort in the neck and shoulders and improved work ability.

Work ability is measured using a self-report questionnaire that combines information on health and medical complaints with information on one's perception of one's own ability to work – for example rating current work ability compared to lifetime best on a scale from 0–10. People scoring highly on work ability are more likely to report that they are closer to their lifetime best at work and have the mental resources to cope.

Most of the volunteers using sit-stand workstations rated the adjustability of the furniture as good (83.3 percent), and 75.0 percent were satisfied with the workstations. About 41.7 percent of the intervention participants, who were exclusively female, used the sit-stand function on a daily basis.

## PHYSICAL ACTIVITY GUIDELINES

At the time of writing, a number of governments have published guidelines for the amount of physical activity needed to maintain health. USA government guidelines recommend at least 150–300 minutes of moderate-intensity aerobic activity per week (brisk walking or fast dancing) and some muscle strengthening activity at least two days per week. Putting this into perspective 150–300 minutes (2.5–5 hours) of brisk walking per week (at about 5 METS) comes to 12.5–25 MET hours. If an office worker spends 40 hours per week sitting (at 1.5 METS or 60 MET hours per week) adding 2.5 hours of physical activity per week by walking briskly to the office gives an increase in the total physical activity (excluding after-hours activity) of 21 percent. Five hours of brisk walking per week gives an increase in physical activity of 42 percent. This may seem a lot but is far below the 124.4 MET hours worked by our fictional 1950s housewife in Chapter 4 which is over 100 percent greater.

Others have proposed more demanding recommendations – for example, Straker and Mathiassen (2009) suggest:

1. To maintain muscle strength: at least 6 repetitions of an exercise to fatigue twice per week.
2. To maintain bone mineral density: at least 10 vertical jumps per day, 3 days per week.
3. To maintain cardiovascular fitness: at least 20 minutes of moderate exercise twice per week).
4. To avoid diseases associated with inactivity: 30 minutes/day of moderate activity.
5. To maintain a healthy weight: 60 minutes of moderate activity per day.

## KEY POINTS

1. Take regular short breaks from sitting.
2. Don't sit still.
3. Sit for no longer than 20 minutes at a time. Five minutes standing for every 15 minutes of sitting seems beneficial.
4. Choose the default. If nudging is a good way to get people to stand more why not choose nonadjustable tables at a height suitable for standing and then provide seats or stools appropriate for work at high tables? This may be more effective (and less expensive) than providing seats suitable for low desks and then providing desks that can be raised for standing.
5. At the time of writing, the evidence seems to suggest that the adverse effects of sedentary work can be mitigated simply by enabling employees

to sit and stand naturally and move around at will – in effect the behaviors described in Chapter 1. At the time of writing, many offices do not enable employees to do so.

6. Several studies have investigated whether sit-stand working can increase productivity in office tasks. Overall, the findings vary. In practice, productivity is affected by many variables other than workstation design therefore it may be unreasonable to expect healthier ways of working to have immediate effects on productivity, or even to expect that productivity would be improved. In the long term, if people remain healthier as they age, the real benefits may become apparent.

7. Standing does have some clear advantages over sitting (Bridger, 2018):
   a. You can reach further when standing than when sitting.
   b. Body weight can be used to move objects.
   c. Standing requires less legroom than sitting.
   d. Standing is safer on moving vehicles that vibrate.
   e. Pressure in the lumbar intervertebral discs is lower when standing.
   f. Standing can be maintained with little muscle activity and requires no attention.
   g. Muscle power of the upper body is twice as great when standing compared to sitting or semi-sitting.

8. The evidence to date indicates that it is not sitting, per se, that is harmful, but the lack of skeletal muscle activity that occurs when seated. It may not be necessary to stand more at work to gain benefits if employees can be more active when sitting at their desks. Products that enable active sitting and their benefits are reviewed in Chapter 8.

# 7 Bad Habits Versus Active Workplaces

Motivation is what gets you started. Habit is what keeps you going.

**Jim Ryun at www.brainyquote.com/topics/habit**

There has been a lot of attention recently in the media and on television about public health issues associated with physical inactivity and the increase in overweight and obesity. One recent initiative concerns "active buildings" to promote a more physically active lifestyle at work. We have already seen that changes to office furniture and layout do sometimes bring about changes in behavior – people do use sit-stand desks when they are available, maybe not standing as much as they should, but the desks do get used.

Many studies show only modest reductions in sitting time, so it seems reasonable to ask whether sitting at work has become a habit? If it has, how do we change it?

In this chapter, we will look at some of the reasons why it is difficult to change from a sedentary lifestyle and what can be done to help.

## WORKPLACE FITNESS PROGRAMS HAVE A LONG HISTORY – OLD HABITS DIE HARD

There is nothing new about workplace fitness programs. Hardman et al. (1989) investigated the effects of a program of brisk walking on a group of sedentary middle-aged women. They followed a progressive regime building up speed after 12 months and averaging 16–17km per week. The women exercised for about 155 minutes per week at approximately 60 percent of their maximal oxygen uptake – at 60 percent of maximum, a person can exercise for about 80 minutes before exhaustion. In Hardman's program, the walking was spread out over the week in several sessions totaling 150 minutes per week. After 12 months, beneficial changes in the ratio of total cholesterol to HDL ("good") cholesterol concentration were observed in the walkers, compared to a control group.

In the 1980s, IBM launched a corporate fitness program "A Plan for Life," which was evaluated by Goetzel et al. (1994). Program participants and non-participants were compared over a five-year period. At the end of five years, program participants were found to have lower risk indices such as total and low density lipoprotein ("bad") cholesterol and smoking. Similar programs have been found to reduce absenteeism when implemented over a three-year period (Knight et al., 1994). Cox et al. (1981) evaluated the effects of an employee fitness program in two Canadian assurance companies. Compared to the control company, participants in the experimental company improved their ability to take up and deliver oxygen to the tissues, reduced their body fat percentage and had more positive attitudes towards their employment. So, the participants in the fitness program were leaner and had better endurance than non-participants.

Given that these programs were shown to be beneficial 30–40 years ago, why have they not been taken up more widely and why has the prevalence of overweight and obesity continued to increase? One reason is that, although the programs were successful, there were costs associated with organizing them, recruiting participants and keeping people interested. If organizations don't support these programs then they won't take place unless employees organize their own programs. That, of course, requires commitment and herein lies *a psychological explanation*.

## SITTING AS A HABIT

People who work in offices are in the "habit of sitting." They sit automatically because that is what they are used to and that is how offices have been designed since the days of the Larkin Building, over 100 years ago. Workstations are designed to enable office workers to carry out their work while seated. For those who are in the habit of sitting all day, to do anything else – go for a walk at lunchtime, use the stairs instead of the lift and so on requires a conscious effort, not just to do something differently, but to remember to do it in the first place!

Busy office workers, already focussed on their daily tasks, may shy away from the effort to change their daily routines or they may just forget to make the changes. Changing one's daily habits requires *self-monitoring* and *self-monitoring requires self-control*.

## SELF-CONTROL AND HABIT FORMATION

Doing familiar things by habit doesn't require as much self-control as not doing them (e.g., eating a chocolate cookie with your morning cup of coffee, as opposed to not eating one, if eating the cookie is what you are used to!). Self-monitoring – paying attention to what you are doing, requires self-control and self-control is a limited resource. When we use it, we use it up, momentarily at least and we spend much of our lives on "automatic pilot," so to speak. Many readers will recall arriving home in the car after a busy day at the office with almost no recollection of the journey home. This is because driving is a well-learned skill, it requires little conscious effort to steer, brake or respond to traffic signals. Under these circumstances, many drivers are more likely to have spent the journey home day-dreaming or reviewing the events of the day and planning for tomorrow than noticing a new advertisement on a billboard at a familiar intersection.

When workload is high, well-learned habits such as driving are insufficient to meet the demands. Automatic pilot isn't enough. Continuing with the driving example; imagine you are driving with a colleague to a business meeting while discussing your joint approach to achieve the desired business outcome. Suddenly, you hear a siren, cars pull over to the side of the road, braking abruptly. You stop talking immediately – all of your attention is required to assess the situation and to make room and be ready for whatever is coming. You pull over and allow three fire engines and an ambulance to pass! As soon as they are gone, the normal flow of traffic is resumed and you resume your conversation. For a moment, you had to react quickly to an unfamiliar situation, assess it and respond in a novel way that was non-habitual. That required conscious effort, leaving no spare capacity to continue your conversation with your colleague.

In order to respond quickly, you had to draw on a set of higher cognitive processes which some researchers refer to as "executive function." According to Banich (2009):

> Various functions and abilities are thought to fall under the rubric of executive function. These include prioritizing and sequencing behavior, inhibiting familiar or stereotyped behaviors, creating or maintaining an idea of what task or information is most relevant to current purposes, providing resistance to information that is distracting or task irrelevant, switching between task goals, utilizing relevant information in support of decision making, categorizing or otherwise abstracting common elements across items and handling novel information or situations.

Acts of self-control – such as not eating a blueberry muffin after lunch and going for a walk outside instead – require executive function. In order to successfully exercise self-control in daily life – or at least long enough to become more active at work, office workers need to monitor their actions in relation to their goals and intentions – to pay attention to what they are doing.

Why is this so difficult and why does it fail so often?

An obvious explanation is that people go to the office to work and not to exercise or to benefit their health in other ways. Office work makes demands on executive function all the time (Semmer et al., 1995). Many office workers have tight deadlines to meet during which they must:

- Resist distraction when carrying out a task (e.g., concentrate on a task when working in a noisy open-plan office)
- Control their own impulses (e.g., refrain from shouting at the computer when the screen freezes in the middle of a critical task)
- Overcome inner resistance (e.g., carry out an unpleasant task or attend a boring meeting when they really don't want to)
- Cope with emotional dissonance (e.g., having to appear friendly and personable to a business rival).

Recent research on self-control indicates that it is a limited resource and that, when it is used, it is used up (for a while, at least). Baumeister et al. (2007) make a straightforward analogy between the strength of our self-control and our muscular strength. Acts of self-control bring about reductions in the ability to carry out further acts of self-control in the same way that short, intense muscular exertions cause temporary drops in strength.

In one experiment (Baumeister et al., 1998) volunteers had to wait in a room before trying to solve (deliberately unsolvable) problems. The experimenters wanted to know whether making people exert self-control beforehand would affect how long they persisted with the unsolvable problems. The key variable of interest was how long the volunteers would persist with the problems before giving up. Outside the waiting room, fresh chocolate cookies were being baked, filling the room with a delicious smell. On the table were plates full of chocolate cookies and radishes (Figure 7.1). One group was told that they were able to eat the cookies and the experimenters checked behind a one-way mirror to see if they did. Another group was told not to eat the cookies but to try the radishes instead (a third group went straight in to solve the problems). It was found that the group that ate the radishes gave up on the problems more quickly than the others. The explanation was that this group had to exert self-control to resist the temptation to eat the cookies whereas the other groups had no demands on self-control (most people are not tempted to eat radishes when there are chocolate cookies on the table, Figure 7.1). Having to exert self-control before attempting the problems had weakened their self-control and so they gave up more quickly.

Following this line of reasoning, it is not surprising that after a hard day at the office, people go home with lower executive control (which is why they can't remember anything about the journey home and didn't notice that the billboard at that familiar intersection had just been changed and was advertising a time-limited discount on one of their favorite vacation venues).

Some common symptoms of mental fatigue after work are (see Sluiter et al. (2003) for more information):

- Trouble concentrating on things after work
- Difficulty showing interest in others
- Wanting to be left alone for a while
- Feeling too tired to start other activities.

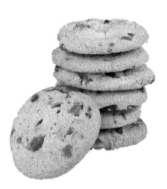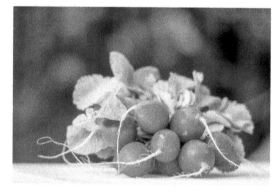

**FIGURE 7.1** Radishes versus chocolate chip cookie? Is self-control a limited resource? Research suggests that resisting temptation lowers our ability to persevere on a task (see text for explanation).

Under these circumstances, despite the best of intentions, old habits die hard. After a tiring day's work, we may know that we should go for a run, eat healthier food or clean the house when we get home, but we cannot overcome our reluctance to do so, nor can we avoid the distraction of our favorite TV show, nor resist the impulse to drink a nice glass of wine.

## SELF-CONTROL AND SUGAR

If Baumeister and his colleagues are right and self-control is a limited resource that gets used up when we use it, several important questions come to mind:

- Why is self-control a limited resource – when we use it, why does it get used up?
- How can we recover self-control?
- How can we develop healthier habits at work so that we don't need to exercise self-control – how can we get active working under the control of the "autopilot"?

Gailliot (2015) summarized the research that suggests that blood glucose levels in the brain affect our ability to exercise self-control. When we *do* exercise self-control, blood glucose levels drop and that lowers the capacity for further acts requiring self-control (such as persisting with the unsolvable problem after resisting the temptation to eat chocolate cookies). This drop in blood glucose levels is not specific to any particular task or activity – as long as the task requires self-control (such as doing mental arithmetic or not drinking wine while preparing dinner) it has the same effect – it reduces resistance and we are more likely to give up.

This explains why office workers, even though they may have sit-stand workstations and even though they know that standing for a while is healthier than sitting all day, may continue to sit because they are absorbed in their work. The mental effort to stop working, stand-up, adjust the desk and maybe the screen as well, is too great.

## RECOVERING SELF-CONTROL

One way to recover self-control according to this view is to drink something high in sugar (preferably glucose). Although there is evidence that glucose drinks can be used to restore self-control, they are not recommended in view of all the evidence in preceding chapters about the links between sedentary lifestyles and the development of health complaints such as Type II diabetes.

Another way of restoring self-control is to do something that does not require it – the glucose levels in the brain are restored automatically. Activities that do not require the executive functions described earlier have the following characteristics:

- You don't have to pay much attention to what you are doing (no self-monitoring needed)

- Your attention is not demanded by a particular task (because you can carry out the task on "autopilot" so to speak)
- No willpower is needed (you don't have to make an effort to carry on with the task because it is enjoyable, interesting or frees the mind to think about other things).

In an experiment by Berman et al. (2008), participants were given a demanding memory task to do in the laboratory. Some of the participants then went for a 50-minute walk in an arboretum and the others for a 50-minute walk in the city. All participants then performed further memory tasks in the lab. It was found that the performance of those who went for a walk in the arboretum was restored more than those who walked in the city. The explanation was that the walk in the arboretum placed fewer demands on attention, allowing the mind to wander, surrounded by non-intrusive stimuli and was therefore restorative. City walkers had to deal with intrusive stimuli, directing their attention to traffic signals, avoiding other pedestrians and so on (Figure 7.2).

The means by which some environments are more restorative than others was described by Kaplan (1995) in his *attention restoration theory*. In much of our daily lives, out attention is directed to meeting the demands at hand – the demands of work, of paying the bills, remembering to fill-up with gas on the drive home from work and so on. When our capacity to direct our attention is limited, the effort to do so increases and we seek refuge in undemanding activities. In Berman's experiment, the walk around the arboretum did not demand the volunteers to direct their attention to anything in particular but was sufficiently rich in stimuli to minimize boredom.

It is ironic perhaps that many recreational sports activities also enable attention to be restored because they make few demands on executive control in *those who participate habitually*. Many runners report experiencing the "runners high" a feeling of "being in the moment," free of the cares of the day. Gym goers also report a feeling of mindfulness when engaged in well-practiced exercise routines. For those who do not exercise this way, getting started requires self-control, which is why they find it difficult to begin and why some never start or give up after the first few attempts.

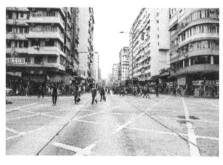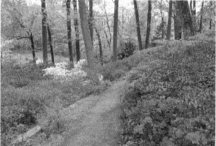

FIGURE 7.2   Promoting recovery – a walk in a crowded city center or in an arboretum. (Source: Pixabay.)

## ACTIVE WORKPLACES AND HEALTHY HABITS

If office workers have to think about moving more at work, then the outlook for reducing sedentary lifestyles in the office isn't good – because office workers will be thinking about work and not about being more active. A more active lifestyle has to become habitual at work if it is to last – office workers will be more active without thinking about it.

A good place to start to follow this line of reasoning is to ask a simple question. Are people who report that physical activity is a habit for them really more active in everyday life? Are people who say that they climb the stairs at work automatically, without thinking, or that they walk to printers or to get coffee automatically, really more active than those who don't report these habits?

Smith et al. (2018) monitored the activity levels of office workers who had completed a questionnaire with items such as:

> Being active in the workplace – (e.g., "walking to printers, for refreshment breaks, to coffee points is something I do automatically, I do without thinking" and "climbing stairs at work is something I do automatically, I do without thinking").

Eighty one percent of the office workers reported being habitually active at work and 62 percent reported climbing stairs habitually. People who reported being active habitually had more "sit-to-stand transitions" at their desks than those who did not report being in the habit, suggesting that the reported habits did reflect a more active lifestyle at work. Interestingly and, perhaps, disappointingly, habit strength for stair climbing was negatively associated with the time spent stepping per hour – which may indicate that stair climbers compensate by sitting more when they get back to their desks!

The activity levels of all the office workers in this study were low, possibly due to the nature of their jobs and the lack of opportunity to be more active. The average step count per hour was 440 – about 3500 steps per day, well below the WHO recommended count of 10,000 steps per day. They spent an average of 15 percent of the time standing and 3 percent of the time walking with an average of just over three sit-stand transitions per hour. These low levels of activity may explain why the reported habits were not more strongly related to physical activity. However, as we saw in Chapter 4, even low levels of activity appear to bring health benefits.

So, if active working habits really do lead to a more active lifestyle at work, how can we develop these habits?

## TRAINING TO USE SIT-STAND WORKSTATIONS

We saw in Chapter 2 that, in the 1940s, the U.S. Navy developed training films for typists that included advice on setting up the workstation and sitting in the chair to be able to operate the typewriter safely and efficiently. Anecdotally, it seems that this kind of training for typists was common at the time in many parts of the world. We also saw that when computer terminals were introduced into offices in the 1980s, most workers weren't even taught how to type.

If sit-stand workstations are introduced into offices, should office workers be trained how to use them and, if so, what should the training be like? A study by Robertson et al. (2012) provides some insights.

Two groups of volunteers spent 19 days in a test of sit-stand workstations. They were trained to carry out the work of online customer service representatives. One group received minimal ergonomic training (little more than the manufacturer's brochure as might be expected when new furniture is delivered to an office). The second group received a training package dealing with how and why good ergonomics is important and the benefits of varying the posture between sitting and standing. In some ways, the first phase of the training resembles that given to the 1940s typists – slides and a video detailing the basic ergonomics principles; four case studies, group debriefings and hands-on practice at workstation adjustment. Six key messages were delivered in the first phase with the emphasis on the importance of posture change (standing and sitting):

1. How to recognize work-related musculoskeletal disorders and workplace risk factors.
2. Understanding the importance of varying work postures.
3. Understanding how to rearrange the workstation to maximize comfort.
4. Recognizing and understanding visual problems (adjusting the screen height and distance, for example) and reducing visual discomfort.
5. Understanding the importance of rest breaks.
6. Knowing how to change work-rest patterns.

The group who received minimal training had a free choice to stand or sit throughout the study. Those who received the first phase of training went on the work for three days with free choice; then for three days with five minutes standing every 50 minutes with reminders and advice; then for three days with 20 minutes standing every 50 minutes with reminders and advice. Both groups spent the last three days standing or sitting at will.

None of the participants in the minimally trained group stood for any length of time throughout the study suggesting that just giving people sit-stand desks is not enough. Training and practice is needed. On the last three days, people in the trained group spent about an hour per day standing and changed posture around three times per day (standing for about 20 minutes at a time on average).

*Not only did the training change behavior – people in the trained group reported less musculoskeletal and visual discomfort and had better job performance.*

## CHOOSING THE DEFAULT

An alternative to training has already been described in the last chapter – "nudging," which was used in a study of sit-stand workstations where the workstations were set to the standing position at the end of the day. When employees arrived in the office in the morning, all the sit-stand workstations were in the standing position so they were more likely to be used this way – people often choose the default because it's easier. So architects and space planners can consider how building layout can be designed to make more active options the default – or at least, easier. For example: stairways and ramps for wheelchair users can be more accessible than the elevators; hard copy mail has to be collected from a central mailroom and is not delivered to the employees at their desks; individual trash cans are removed from desks so that employees have to take their waste paper to a central office recycling bin; meetings are held in a different part of the building so attendees have to walk; smokers have to leave the building to smoke and so on.

The same nudging principles apply to eating!

## THE OBESOGENIC WORKPLACE

This is not a book about nutrition and the author is not a dietitian. However, designing workplaces to encourage employees to eat a healthier diet is compatible with encouraging them to be more active. You might say they are two sides of the same coin.

Throughout history, human populations have survived on a wide variety of diets and *Homo sapiens* is a highly adaptable omnivore (Shorland, 1988). Evidence from the remains of bones in caves indicates that *Homo erectus* survived on a diet that was 70 percent meat (mainly venison). However, in common with modern hunter-gathering tribes, it is unlikely that they were able to hunt a sufficient quantity of game to cause a Stone Age obesity epidemic! Further, the fat content of wild game is lower than in modern domesticated animals as is the fat content of marine mammals and fish that form a large part of the diet of modern Inuit. Indeed for most of recorded history, from ancient Greece and Rome to modern times, people have subsisted on cereals such as barley and millet supplemented with small amounts of olives, cheese, figs and beans. The Western "meat-milk" diet of the last 100 years is relatively new and has had two effects on human populations. This first was to cause an increase in stature as previously undernourished populations were then able to grow to their genetic potential. This was closely followed by an increase in over-weight and obesity due to sedentary lifestyles and an abundance of cheap, processed foods far denser in calories than naturally occurring ("wild") foods.

Lunch is a product of the Industrial Revolution. Factories were often too far from employees' homes for them to go home for lunch so it soon became apparent to factory owners and builders that workers had to eat lunch to have energy for the afternoon shift and that they needed somewhere to eat it. For many low paid workers, lunch would be the main meal of the day.

The Larkin Building had a staff canteen on the top floor.

Most office workers in the internet age enjoy "super-nutrition" in the form of a wide variety and abundance of calorie-dense foods. Apart from an excess of calories, the modern diet can also be nutritionally distorted due to the removal of naturally occurring but beneficial components such as bran and other residues to make white flour and the addition of other components such as salt. "Low fat" products in which fats have been removed may have added sugar to restore some flavor. Because insulin is a "fat-sparing" hormone, the sugar is absorbed into the tissues and used as an energy source, instead of fat being used as an energy source.

## NUTRITIONAL "NUDGES" TO A HEALTHIER DEFAULT

Are modern offices "obesogenic"? Does working in an office make you gain weight? Not necessarily, but we have already reviewed some of the evidence that a sedentary lifestyle is harmful and that it is beneficial to increase one's level of physical activity. One of the ways to make office work healthier is to design offices so that office workers spend less time sitting.

Although we can't tell office workers what to eat, we can make healthier options more salient and available and we can introduce a little "friction" so that unhealthy options are less accessible. For example:

1. Provide accessible facilities for food storage and preparation (refrigerator, microwave) for those wishing to bring their own food
2. Offer healthier (and inexpensive) food options in the staff canteen
3. Make healthier (i.e., lower in calories, higher in other nutrients such as vitamins) food options more available than unhealthier options (e.g., salads on display in the buffet, fries have to be requested in advance)
4. Better nutritional information on prepared food products
5. Healthier food options in vending machines
6. Discourage eating lunch at the desk – proper break-out areas for lunch
7. Workplace incentives for obesity prevention programs
8. Work-scheduling to allow a proper lunch break.

## FROM WORKPLACE FITNESS TO WELL-BUILDINGS

A number of more recent developments are Fitwell Certification and the Well-Building Standard®. The focus of both of these initiatives is on the built environment rather than the occupants. Buildings can be certified by scoring their design features in relation to the impact on health and wellbeing of the occupants. The scope is wide and beyond the focus of this book, but it takes many aspects of the environment into account such as air quality, water, nourishment, light, comfort etc.

The Fitwell Workplace Scorecard has 60 items dealing with a range of features of the built environment. Some examples of Fitwell features of buildings are given below. Buildings score highly if:

- A public transport stop is available within 800 meters of the building entrance.
- Showers with lockers are available for regular occupants.
- There is secure and covered bicycle parking within 100 feet or 30 meters of a building entrance for a minimum of 5 percent of regular occupants or exceeding demand as dictated by an occupant survey by 1 percent.
- Permanent fitness equipment in outdoor spaces is accessible to all regular occupants.
- There is an accessible stairwell equally or more visible than any elevators and/or escalators from the main building entrance.
- There are permanent point-of-decision signs promoting stair use at elevator call areas.

- A tobacco-free building policy has been implemented.
- Access to sufficient active workstations is provided.
- There are views of nature from a majority of workspaces.
- There are common break areas accessible to all regular occupants to accommodate lunchtime activity.
- A dedicated exercise room accessible free of charge for all regular occupants is provided.
- Healthy food choices are encouraged through pricing incentives.

## A WORD OF CAUTION

Health behaviors are difficult to change and the improvements resulting from public health campaigns are often small. In a recent review of studies to improve diet and physical activity, Hutchinson and Wilson (2012) concluded that most interventions aimed at improving diet and/or exercise yielded small benefits on a range of health measures. They also cited a famous study by Crum and Langer (2007) who compared a group of hotel room attendants who were told that their work was good exercise with another group who were not told that it was good exercise. After four weeks, the first group had lowered their body mass index (BMI), percentage body fat and lower systolic blood pressure whereas the second group had not. One way of understanding these results is by comparing them to the "placebo effect" in medicine. Merely establishing a positive mindset seems to be beneficial. Hutchinson and Wilson found that the most successful intervention studies seemed to be those that used motivational methods, such as the use of rewards or incentives, and focussed on changing only one thing at a time rather than trying to improve everything at once (diet or exercise, but not both at once).

A more recent review by Shaw et al. (2019) found that there was a shortage of good studies but there was some evidence that diet can be improved by environmental interventions. The interventions that appear to work best include: reducing barriers to healthier eating; increasing the opportunities for and availability of healthy options; and restricting the availability of less healthy options.

These findings report modest benefits and are consistent with some of the research on sit-stand workstations reviewed in earlier chapters – although office workers will use them, the time spent standing is usually small compared to the time spent sitting. However, we have also seen that even modest changes towards more activity can be beneficial over long periods of time. The apparent superiority of motivational approaches to behavior change suggests that when introducing new facilities we should focus on the benefits of change rather than the dis-benefits or risks of not changing.

Several authors (e.g., Brownell, 2011) have called for a "benign paternalism" in which, for example, a "soda tax" is added to the price of sugary beverages to offset the high health costs of obesity and this is being seriously discussed in some countries. Whether employers should take a similar approach and ban the sale of such products on their premises in the same way that tobacco and alcohol are often banned in the workplace is open to debate.

## KEY POINTS

1. Consider the training requirements when introducing initiatives to encourage more active working. Training in office ergonomics and correct adjustment of sit-stand workstations should cover both the benefits of varying posture ("why") and the knowledge to adjust workstations correctly ("how").

2. Remembering to be more active in the office requires self-control and self-control requires that we direct our attention internally. In the office, however, our attention is directed externally to the tasks at hand. Once active working becomes habitual, self-control is no longer needed and active working becomes habitual.

3. Build movement into sedentary jobs:
   a. Encourage users of sit-stand desks to stand after lunch
   b. Site catering facilities away from the office
   c. Hold meetings at standing desks after lunch
   d. Discourage employees from eating at their desks
   e. Encourage more use of the stairs.

4. Encourage the development of new habits:
   a. Remove barriers to healthy alternatives (e.g., provide proper storage facilities for bicycles for those wishing to cycle to work and showers for those wishing to exercise at lunchtime).
   b. Select tasks to carry out only when standing – speaking on the phone, reading hard copy, sorting papers are examples.

5. Make the workplace less obesogenic:
   a. Provide simple facilities for food storage and preparation (refrigerator, microwave) for those wishing to bring their own food.
   b. Provide healthier (and inexpensive) food options in the staff canteen.
   c. Make healthier food options more available (e.g., salads on display in the buffet, fries have to be requested in advance)
   d. Provide better nutritional information on prepared food products
   e. Have healthier food options in vending machines
   f. Discourage eating lunch at the desk – provide proper break-out areas for lunch
   g. Schedule time away from the desk to engage in obesity prevention programs
   h. Adjust work-scheduling to allow proper lunch breaks.

6. Make default options for simple tasks more active:
   a. Stairways, ramps for wheelchair users can be more accessible than the elevators
   b. Hard copy mail has to be collected from a central mailroom and is not delivered to employees at their desks
   c. Individual trash cans are removed from desks so that employees have to take their waste paper to a central office recycling bin
   d. Smokers have to leave the building to smoke.

7. If you think you spend too much time sitting down, try to create some new habits around standing up (e.g., move your phone to the other side of the desk so you have to get up to use it; park at the far end of the car park rather than close to the entrance to the building and so on).

# 8 Choosing Products for Active Office Work

The affordances of the environment are what it offers the animal, what it provides or furnishes, either for good or ill. The verb to afford is found in the dictionary, the noun affordance is not. I have made it up. I mean by it something that refers to both the environment and the animal in a way that no existing term does. It implies the complementarity of the animal and the environment.

**Gibson (1979, p. 127)**

Do workplace interventions for reducing sitting at work do any good?

A recent review by an international group known as the "Cochrane Collaboration" evaluated the effects of workplace interventions to reduce sitting at work (Shrestha et al., 2015). The Cochrane Collaboration is an international network of scientists and medical experts who review the current state of knowledge about the effectiveness of healthcare interventions using strict, but widely accepted, criteria to come to some conclusions about the strength of the evidence in favor. The Cochrane Reviewers do this by reviewing all published scientific papers in an area, filtering out those reports that are of poor quality and assessing those that are left.

What did they find? Out of the many studies that have been carried out, the reviewers found only eight studies of sufficient quality for further review – involving a total of 1125 volunteers. Six of the trials evaluated the effects of sit-stand desks; two evaluated computer prompting and one the effect of walking during breaks. Overall, the strength of the evidence in favor of any of these interventions was weak and sometimes inconsistent. For sit-stand desks, there was evidence for a reduction in sitting time of 113 minutes per day but the evidence was weak.

These findings, taken at face value, are not encouraging. It should be remembered though that scientifically sound studies of reducing sitting time at work are difficult to conduct – particularly over long periods of time and using large numbers of volunteers. Perhaps more time is needed to demonstrate the benefits?

There is a more obvious explanation as to why interventions to reduce sitting at work have yielded only modest results. The alternative to sitting in most office jobs is standing. Most office workers spend a great deal of the day at their computers or laptops and would have to stand very still. As we saw in earlier chapters, standing still is unnatural, uncomfortable and unhealthy. Maybe new design ideas are needed to permit office workers to increase their physical activity naturally and comfortably while still being able to work efficiently?

## REQUIREMENTS FOR AN ACTIVE
## WORKSPACE FOR OFFICE WORKERS

What would an ideal dynamic workspace for office workers look like? There is no simple answer to this question because what the workspace will consist of and what it will look like will depend on the creativity of the designer and the task requirements the workspace must meet.

In 1994, a group of human factors specialists, industrial designers and design students met in Cape Town to discuss these issues and to define the requirements for an ideal prototype standing workspace (Bridger et al., 1994). Starting from first principles, they came up with the following key requirements:

- Only parts of the body are supported at any time
- Only part of the weight is relieved
- Left-right weight shift and interchange of posture is permitted
- Continuous variation of posture is the starting point in design
- It is assumed that the stander has a continuous desire to change posture.

In order for office workers to stand and move more naturally at work, even at an "ideal" active workstation, there are two key considerations that have to do with the way we interact with our surroundings. Both of these considerations follow from the previous chapter and were considered to be habit formation and the mental demands of daily life.

If the aim is to be more active at work, we can try "nudging" people to become more active (making it easier to be more active) and use "friction" to reduce inactivity (making it more difficult to sit still all day). In order for these tactics to work, the office environment and the furniture have to be designed to encourage activity – to provide *affordances* for activity and for movement.

"Affordances" are characteristics of spaces that encourage certain behaviors. For example, a footrail at the bar in a pub provides the "affordance" of changing foot position and weight distribution while "propping-up the bar."

In Figure 8.1 we can see a shop owner talking to a customer. Notice the shop owner's right shin is resting on a stool. The stool provides the "affordance" for the posture even though that is not the stool's main function. Alongside the photograph, we can see a concept drawing of a standing desk that provides the same affordance while working at the desk. The desk has been designed to make it more likely that employees will change posture when standing – the affordance to do so is part of the design.

How about walking while we work? Many people walk and send or read text messages at the same time in their daily lives. A laboratory study by Hinton et al. (2018)

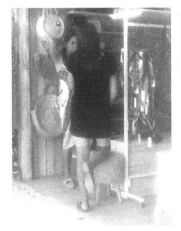 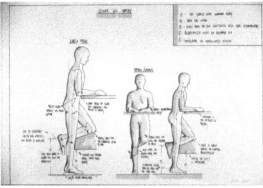

**FIGURE 8.1** Shop owner adopting a natural standing posture while dealing with a customer. In the second figure, a concept design for a workstation that provides the "affordance" for this kind of posture.

looked at walking patterns and texting performance of students walking in treadmills. It seems that as long as neither task is too demanding, people are able to do both simultaneously.

## TREADMILL DESKS

McEwan et al. (2015) reviewed research on treadmill desks (Figure 8.2) and identified a number of benefits:

1. Reductions in total and LDL cholesterol in overweight and obese volunteers and an increase in HDL ("good") cholesterol over nine months using treadmill desks.
2. Reductions in blood pressure and evidence of better glucose control in volunteers with high blood pressure when they started using treadmill desks.
3. Improved blood glucose response in overweight participants using a treadmill desk for two minutes for every ten minutes of sitting.
4. Some evidence that using a treadmill desk for nine months to one year brings about significant weight loss and reductions in waist circumference, particularly in obese volunteers.
5. Walking on a treadmill at 1.6km/h or at a self-selected speed does not appear to affect typing performance.
6. Although the findings of different studies are mixed, walking at 1.6km/h seems best if task performance is to be maintained. Different studies do not always agree and there is evidence for learning effects as performance improves after several months using a treadmill desk – people get used to "walking while they work."

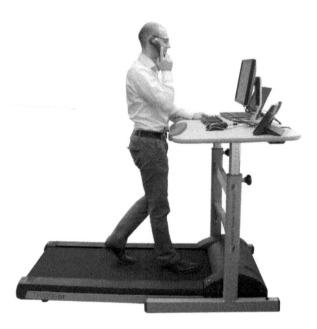

**FIGURE 8.2** A treadmill desk providing the affordance of walking while you work. (Source: Courtesy of TNO, dep. Healthy Living, the Netherlands.)

7. Walking slowly on a treadmill does not appear to affect cognitive performance. This is not surprising since such walking is likely to be unobtrusive and will not distract the user from the task at hand.
8. In general, use of treadmill desks in the office can bring health benefits, more so than standing desks because the physical activity of walking is greater (2–3 METS for walking compared to 1–2 for standing).

Before considering the use of treadmill desks in offices, it should be remembered that, because energy expenditure is greater when using treadmill desks than when sitting, treadmill users may find a lower office temperature more acceptable – about 2.7 degrees Celsius lower according to Gao et al. (2018). A single temperature setting in spaces with active workstations may not satisfy all occupants, thus providing personal temperature control to keep employees comfortable might be necessary.

## PEDAL DESKS

Pedal desks (Figure 8.3) seem to bring similar benefits in increased energy expenditure to treadmill desks. Schuna et al. (2019) compared energy expenditure of eight male and eight female volunteers while: sitting at rest; seated in an office chair typing; typing while seated on a pedal desk at their own pace; typing on a treadmill desk while walking at their own pace. Energy expenditure when using the pedal and treadmill desks was about double that when typing seated at a conventional desk, although the energy expenditure of males was higher on the treadmill desk than at the pedal desk.

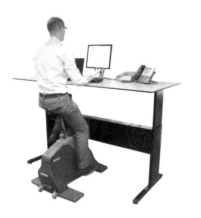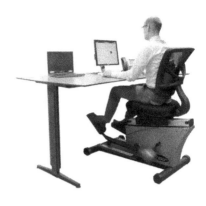

**FIGURE 8.3**   A pedal desk providing the affordance of cycling at your desk.

In a separate study, Proença et al. (2018) investigated the acceptability of a pedal desk – the Pennington Pedal Desk – when 42 full-time sedentary workers carried out a variety of tasks including searching the internet and composing an email. They then rated the acceptability of the desk on a five point rating scale. The volunteers in the study indicated that they would use the desk daily (median expected time of use was four hours per day) and most were confident that they could type proficiently when using the desk. Participants pedaled at an average rate of 54.8 RPM (just under one revolution per second) raising the activity level by an additional 1 to 2 METS (estimated).

## MAKING SITTING MORE ACTIVE: FIDGET DEVICES AND "CORE" CHAIRS

We reviewed evidence in Chapter 6 that even short breaks from sitting can be beneficial because they require additional muscle activity and that the activity has a variety of benefits – improving blood flow and activating the venous pump. Fidget devices, such as the "foot-fidget" in Figure 8.4, are designed to enable people to move more while sitting at a desk.

They provide an "affordance" for fidgeting.

The "foot-fidget" is an elasticated footrest that fits under the desk of a seated or standing employee. The feet rest on an elasticized central footpad on two flexible cords that run through the tube and attach to the four upright legs on the stand. Users are able to "bounce" their feet on the device.

Koepp et al. (2016) evaluated a fidget device to determine whether its use would increase the energy expenditure of sedentary employees. Volunteers in their study worked by using the internet and checking emails for short periods of time. First, they sat on a conventional office chair, then after 20 minutes were given the fidget device to use for 20 minutes. Following this, the conventional chair was changed for a "core" chair designed to encourage movement of the upper body (Figure 8.5). They then followed some chair-based exercise videos and went for a 20-minute walk at about 3.2km/h. This procedure enabled the researchers to compare the size of any

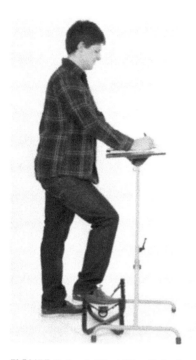
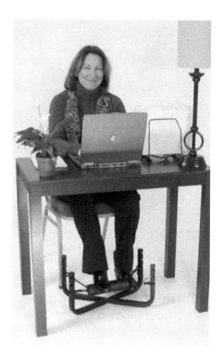

**FIGURE 8.4** A "foot-fidget" device providing the affordance of fidgeting at your desk. (Source: courtesy of Classroom seating solutions, www.footfidget.com.)

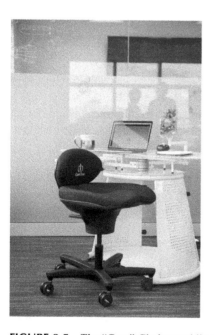
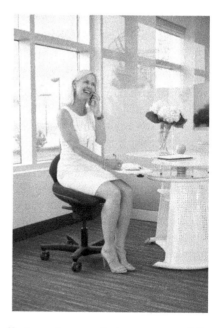

**FIGURE 8.5** The "Core" Chair providing the affordance for upper body movement while seated. (Source: courtesy of CoreChair Inc, www.corechair.com.)

effects on energy expenditure and heart rate of the fidget device and the core chair with the effects of walking and chair-based exercises.

Compared to sitting on the conventional chair, the core chair increased energy expenditure by 20 percent, with no effect on heart rate; the fidget device increased energy expenditure by 30 percent with no increase in heart rate; the desk-based exercises doubled energy expenditure and increased heart rate to similar levels observed when walking at 3.2km/h.

Several other studies on "core" chairs have been carried out. The chair has a very low backrest which acts to stabilize the pelvis of the sitter which encourages the use of the "core" musculature of the trunk and legs to maintain postural stability. Further, because the low backrest does not impede movement of the upper body, it provides the *affordance* for movement compared to conventional high-back computer chairs that provide the affordance for reclining. Cheema et al. (2017) carried out a small study comparing the "core" chair with a conventional chair during four hours of sedentary work. Some differences between the "core" chair and the conventional chair were found and these included: increased movement of the trunk when the core chair was used; decreased sensitivity of the heels suggesting that more use was made of the legs to stabilize the body; calf circumference increased over the four hours when both chairs were used but there was evidence for a smaller increase when the "core" chair was used. The experimenters also gave the subjects a cognitive test to do at the beginning and end of the four-hour period. Subjects were more likely to make "errors of commission" (hitting a key in response to a stimulus appearing on the computer screen, when the correct response was to ignore the stimulus) on both chairs, but the increase was lower with the core chair.

From a practical point of view, although the core chair and foot-fidget did not increase energy expenditure as much as exercising or walking, the benefits can be obtained without interrupting work. Further, although the researchers did not make this claim themselves, the increase in energy expenditure when using the fidget device was probably greater than that observed when people stand still. So, one conclusion that can be drawn from this study is that it is not necessary to stand to increase energy expenditure as long as the design of the sedentary workspace provides the *affordance* for movement and there may be some benefits for work performance as people who move more when sitting are likely to be more alert.

## EXERCISE BALLS

Large, inflatable balls have long been used in clinical physical therapy and, more recently, have been proposed as seats for office workers – particularly office workers who suffer backache when sitting at their desks (Figure 8.6). The rationale for the use of the ball as a seat is twofold: firstly, because the seat bones ("ischial tuberosities") sink into the inflated surface of the ball, they are readily stabilized (Hart, 1998); secondly, the very instability of the ball itself is thought to provide mild, dynamic stimulation of the trunk postural muscles (in particular, the core stability muscles that cross the pelvis) such that constant, slight oscillation in pressure and load values delay the onset of muscle fatigue and discomfort. It is likely that effective stabilization of the pelvis at the ischial tuberosities minimizes the need for compensatory muscular stabilization at the next level up the kinetic chain – the low back. In other words, if you stabilize the pelvis properly, the back muscles have to do less work to maintain the posture of the upper body. Further, because the ball is unstable, small postural muscle changes have to be made by different muscle groups providing frequent, short work and rest periods for different muscle groups.

Is this true? A study by Gregory et al. (2006) compared subjects sitting on an exercise ball for one hour and on a conventional chair for one hour when carrying out computer-based tasks. Very few differences were observed between the ball and the chair in terms of muscle activation or sitting posture. The main difference that was reported was increased discomfort when sitting on the ball! Similar findings were reported by McGill et al. (2006) who suggested that the discomfort when using the ball is due to soft tissue compression. Furthermore, the evidence seems to indicate that the energy expenditure when sitting on an exercise ball is about the same as when sitting on a conventional chair.

Bridger et al. (2000) carried out a trial to compare conventional office chairs with exercise balls and the "kneeling" chairs described in an earlier chapter. Fifty four female secretarial workers volunteered to participate in the study, all of whom complained of back pain lasting several years or more (Figure 8.6). They were interviewed about their back problems and rated body discomfort on diagrams of the body to indicate the location and severity of any pain. All the workspaces of the volunteers were adjusted by the researchers to ensure that the layout met the statutory requirements for work with display screen equipment. This was done to control for factors other than seating that might cause discomfort.

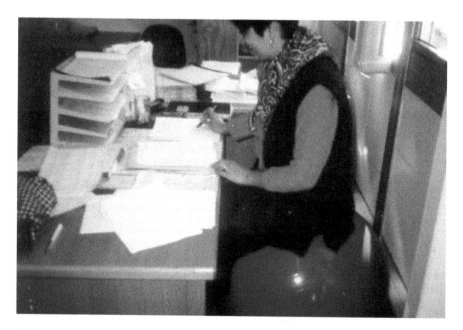

**FIGURE 8.6** Large physiotherapy exercise ball being used as a seat (from the study of Bridger et al. (2000)). The affordance to "wobble while you work."

Participants were then randomly allocated to one of three groups. In the control group, their existing chairs were examined and correctly adjusted by the researchers so that the lumbar supports would provide the correct support for the lumbar spine. The seat height was correctly adjusted in relation to the keyboard and desktop. All control group participants were issued with identical footrests with a 15-degree slope and shown how to use them (no subjects already used a footrest). All control group participants were trained at their desks in the correct techniques for sitting down in the chair to benefit from the lumbar support (see Figure 3.12).

Participants in the experimental groups received either a kneeling chair or an exercise ball. The experimenters demonstrated the use of the seats to the participants at their desks and familiarized them in the use of the devices before the trial commenced. After three weeks, subjects were interviewed again and completed the body diagrams. Data on the usability of the seats and participants' likes and dislikes about them were obtained during the de-briefing session.

There were statistically significant reductions in low back pain for participants in using the kneeling chair and the ball but not for the conventional chair. Perhaps the most interesting finding was the variability in the way the participants responded to the changes. Despite the overall significant reductions in low back pain in the ball and the kneeling chair groups, there was a distinct tendency for these devices to be associated with a worsening of pain in some participants – the spread of pain scores in both groups was much larger at the end of the trial than at the beginning – *so alternative seats aren't for everyone and whether or not an alternative seat is "good for the back" depends on what's wrong in the first place.*

An unanticipated ergonomic problem with both the kneeling chair and the ball was the amount of space they took up. Participants also complained about the tendency for the ball to roll away when not being sat on!

## "CHAIRLESS" CHAIRS

Chairless chairs are passive exoskeletons that enable the wearer to work in standing, semi-standing and sitting positions (Figure 8.7). They provide the affordance of postural change in spaces where there is no furniture or where the furniture is unsuitable for a particular posture.

At the time of writing, there is little peer-reviewed literature on these devices although Luger et al. (2019) report favorably on the comfort of these devices when used in short-term trials.

## DOES ACTIVE WORK DEGRADE MENTAL PERFORMANCE?

The human brain uses a great deal of the energy consumed by the body – at 2 percent of body mass, it uses 20 percent of the energy we consume. Tasks requiring mental effort appear to be those that are most dependent on glucose, the brain's source of energy. If we are carrying out mental work in the office while working on a treadmill, will the treadmill walking degrade our mental ability?

There is evidence that physical tasks can degrade short-term memory (like remembering a new phone number). Scholey et al. (2013) presented people with

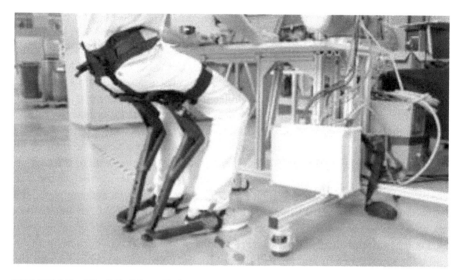

**FIGURE 8.7**   The "Chairless Chair," a wearable exoskeleton to support the body in semi-standing and sitting provides the affordance to sit without a chair. (Source: courtesy of Chairless Chair®, noonee AG, Switzerland.)

a list of 40 words for two seconds each at one second intervals. When a second task was introduced (alternating hand movements of the "fist, chop, slap" kind, in sequence with the words) recall of the words was degraded compared to perform-ing the memory task on its own. Scholey at al. interpreted their findings using the glucose hypothesis. The administration of glucose ten minutes prior to the memory task improved performance of the task when it was effortful (made more difficult by the addition of a concurrent hand movement task) compared to the administra-tion of a placebo (artificially sweetened). However, the beneficial effect of glucose was only apparent when the memory task was made effortful by the inclusion of the secondary task. These data indicate that two seemingly different tasks can interfere with each other by drawing on a common resource – so walking on a treadmill at work might interfere with our ability to do mental tasks if the mental tasks are difficult.

Exercise uses the brain's limited physiological resources due to the large and sustained activation of neural and sensory systems. Brain areas not essential to per-forming the exercise, such as those parts of the frontal lobes which are concerned with higher cognitive functioning, are temporarily inhibited (Dietrich and Sparling, 2004). So, exercising hard on a treadmill or pedal desk might interfere with the performance of even relatively easy mental tasks.

These findings are in agreement with the research on treadmill desks that seems to suggest that we can maintain performance when the activity is relatively mild – 3km/h or about 2–3 METS.

There is some evidence that the active workstations that raise energy expenditure can interfere with tasks requiring fine motor control – using a mouse for example – but the effects are not large (Commissaris et al., 2014, 2016).

## THE ACTIVE TRIANGLE – GETTING THE MIX RIGHT

The evidence suggests that if we want office workers to increase their energy expenditure at work, then active workstations have a role to play. These workstations would seem best for employees with clearly defined tasks at fixed workstations. Getting the mix right would appear to depend on three sets of variables: the workstation itself and the kind of activity it affords, the increase in energy expenditure when active and the demands of the task (Figure 8.8).

Exercise balls, sit-stand workstations and fidget devices do not appear to raise energy expenditure compared to sitting at conventional desks. However, they do have other benefits – greater comfort if used correctly and improved circulation. Dupont et al. (2019) reviewed the evidence for the benefits and possible dis-benefits of cycling workstations, treadmill desks and standing workstations. These are summarized as follows:

- Compared to standing, treadmill desks increase energy expenditure by about 1 MET when walking slowly (see Figure 3.12).
- Cycling workstations also increase energy expenditure by about 1–3 METS depending on the speed of cycling.
- Compared to standing workstations, people using treadmill desks or cycle workstations report higher *perceived exertion* (they report that they are making more of an effort). Perceived exertion is often measured on a 10-point scale where "1" indicates no exertion and "10" indicates maximum exertion. For standing, the effort score was just below "1" on average and 1.74 to 2.6 for treadmill desks and cycling workstations respectively. Effort was perceived to be higher but not high (less than 3/10). So, people report greater effort with these workstations compared to standing but the effort is still very low and unlikely to affect concentration.
- There is some evidence that using a treadmill desk reduces the perceived speed and accuracy of using a mouse and that typing speeds are slightly reduced when using treadmill desks and cycling workstations but again, these differences are small amounting to reductions of only a few words per minute.

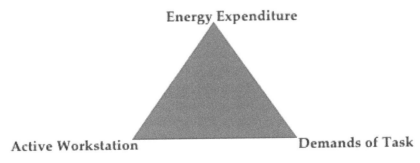

**FIGURE 8.8**  The "Active Triangle" – deciding how to provide the affordance for increased activity at a workplace may mean trading off the requirements of the role against the desired increase in energy expenditure.

- There is some evidence that people feel more alert using treadmill desks and cycling workstations compared to standing and are less bored. There appear to be no effects of working at a treadmill desk or cycling workstation on attention and short-term memory compared to standing.

So, for tasks requiring highly accurate use of the mouse and keyboard, treadmill desks might not be the answer and a seated workstation with fidget bar might be a better workstation alternative if the rest of the office layout encourages more activity, such as walking. For jobs with varying demands involving multiple task objects and requiring reaching and moving, a standing or sit-stand desk might be better. For tasks requiring concentration but not requiring fine control of the mouse or a fast typing speed, treadmill desks and cycling workstations may be appropriate. A lot depends on the scope for redesigning offices and jobs to build more movement away from the desk throughout the day.

## SHORT-TERM VERSUS LONG-TERM BENEFITS

Many new products may seem to have a positive impact when they are introduced and soon after. These effects may not be enduring because they may only be a response to the novelty of the new product. The "Novelty Effect" is well known in experimental research – new products when introduced have a positive impact because they are novel, not because they are better (Bridger, 2018). The novelty creates interest, diverts attention from problems and may even improve performance. New office furniture may lead to a reduction in complaints as office workers experiment with it and adapt themselves to the change. Once the novelty wears off, everything returns to normal and the problems reappear. In the study by Garrett et al. (2019) discussed in Chapter 6, for example, office workers increased the time they stood at their sit-stand workstations when prompted to do so by the software on their laptops. However, the average number of transitions (sit-stand changes) per day, decreased over a three-month period.

Novelty effects may be less likely in situations where change is common. As far as new products are concerned, most of the research at the time of writing shows short-term benefits – whether these will be maintained over long periods of time is unknown.

## KEY POINTS

1. New products are available to increase the activity levels of deskbound workers. They do this in different ways and the benefits are likely to vary. It is unlikely that there is a "one size fits all" solution.
2. Before investing in new designs and new products, it might be best to define the problem that the new initiative is intended to solve and then consider the kinds of solutions that might be worth pursuing.
3. There is evidence that many of the new design ideas for making office work more active are likely to be beneficial – that is, beneficial overall, in general and on the short to medium term. As was seen in the study on

the exercise ball, the extent to which any particular individual will benefit from a particular product is unknown. We saw in an earlier chapter that people experience back pain for different reasons and there can be no "one size fits all" approach to making sedentary work more active.

4. There is evidence that these new design concepts are *efficacious* – they are likely to work *in principle*. Whether they work in real offices for long periods of time and provide a real return on investment – whether they are *effective* – is unknown at the time of writing.

5. Apart from active workstations, designers and managers have many more options for increasing physical activity at work. New buildings can be designed to encourage more use of the stairs and function rooms and cafeterias can be distanced so that employees have to leave their desks as part of normal office work. Job rotation or job enlargement can be used to create new jobs that are more active.

# 9 The Future of Office Work?

The default mode of interacting with a computer is via a monitor sitting in front of a desk … A key concern is determining how to design shared information spaces that provide the right set of physical affordances that will allow people to feel comfortable and know how to interact in the space, which in turn will support the flow of attention across multiple representations and the necessary coordination when collaborating.

**Rogers and Rodden (2002)**

Products such as laptops and cell-phones and the connectivity provided by the internet provide the affordances for mobile working. Much work can now be done at any location that supports the operation of these devices and their use. As I write this paragraph, I am in the middle of the Bay of Biscay, sitting in the lounge of a ferry travelling from the UK to Santander in Spain.

Old ideas about efficiency, where employees sat at their desks all day, date from the days of the Larkin Building and the management philosophy that drove office design in the last century. It is arguable that this philosophy was appropriate at the time – unlike modern laptops and cell-phones, typewriters were bulky and telephones were connected to power sources – so most employees who used these devices had to sit at fixed workstations. The physical design of the office around the time of the Larkin Building afforded the opportunity for efficient performance of office tasks using the technology available at the time. The large, open spaces also afforded management with the ability to supervise employees as they worked.

This way of working is unlikely to be appropriate for future office work in view of the demographic changes that have occurred in the last 100 years and the new technologies and tools that are available. These tools provide affordances for completely different ways of working. These affordances are embedded in the technology used to do the work – the software and the applications on laptops and phones provide the structured environment that affords the opportunity for productive work – rather than the physical layout of the office itself. It is not surprising then, that the number one requirement of office workers when visiting an unfamiliar office is Wi-Fi.

If the affordances for productive work are now embedded in mobile, interconnected devices and people can work almost anywhere, do we still need offices? Maybe, but the places where work is done, either virtual or real, will be designed to provide other kinds of affordances – social and environmental – to support the jobs of the future. Other affordances, unexpected and unplanned, may simply emerge as office design changes. Sit-stand desks set at standing height as the default might provide improved affordances for informal co-working because colleagues passing by will be at the same level as the faces and screens of their standing co-workers thereby facilitating communication (see Figure 9.1).

## ANOTHER DAY AT THE "COFFICE"

Some have suggested that the coffee house of the 17th and 18th centuries may be making a comeback in the form of cafes and other social spaces where people can meet. These are called "third places" (the first is the home, the second is the workplace etc.). In discussing the city as an office, Nenonen et al. (2016) describe the requirements for these third places in terms of accessibility, access, the digital platform, privacy and opportunities for relaxation and interaction that would make them attractive to users (Figure 9.2).

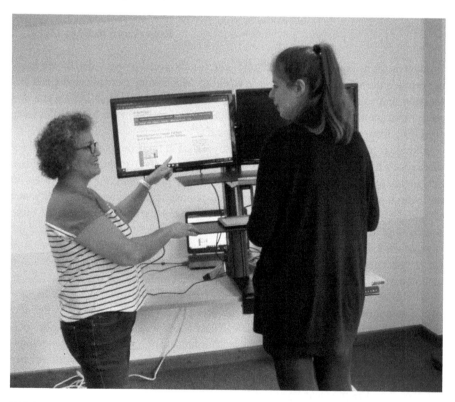

**FIGURE 9.1**    Will stand-biased workstations provide improved affordances for informal co-working?

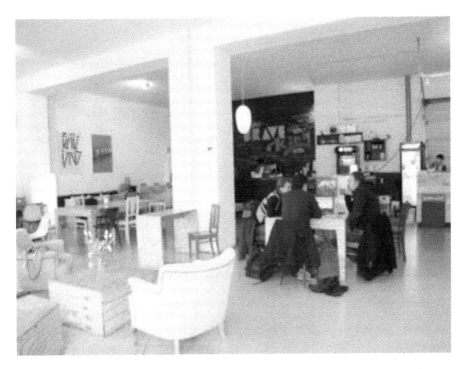

**FIGURE 9.2**   The Office of the Future? The technology provides the affordances for pro-ductive work while the "third place" provides social and other affordances for meeting and networking. (Source: image courtesy of Inka Sankari Tampere University, Finland.)

Nicola Millard of the British Telecom Research and Innovation Centre in the United Kingdom has coined the term "Coffice" to describe these third places. "Shoulder bag workers" go to hubs where they can collaborate and meet others face to face. Social interaction and co-working at these hubs is facilitated by company, coffee and cake!

Offices of the future will need to provide many other kinds of affordances – not just those needed to promote a physically healthy work environment. Social affor-dances, as yet unspecified will be needed for privacy when privacy is needed and for collaborative working in teams – including teams with members participating remotely. These matters are beyond the scope of the present book, but suffice to say, traditional offices have been around for a long time and were originally designed to support work using completely different technologies, whereas the offices of the future will use technologies not yet invented. The optimal design of future offices may well be quite different from the offices of today.

## THE AFFORDANCE WORKSPACE

A futuristic view of the office can be seen in the affordance workspace developed by Dutch architects RAAAF and the artist Barbara Visser (Figure 9.3). This office has no chairs or desks only geometric surfaces varying in angle and tilt, where

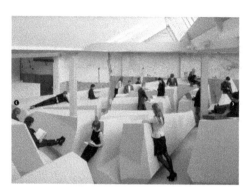
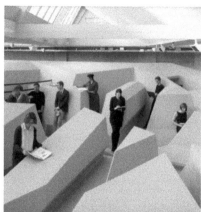

**FIGURE 9.3**   The end of sitting. Concept design for an affordance workspace supporting natural and spontaneous postural behaviors as described in Chapter 1. (Source: Photographs courtesy of RAAAF architects (Rietveld Architecture Art Affordances). Concept design by RAAAF architects and artist Barbara Visser.

employees are able to adopt a variety of postures while working. In many ways, this concept takes us back to Chapter 1 because it provides the affordances for spontaneous postural behavior in a quasi-naturalistic setting.

According to the architects Ronald and Erik Rietveld, the two founders of RAAAF.

> We have developed a concept wherein the chair and desk are no longer unquestionable starting points. … Instead, the installation's various affordances solicit visitors to explore different standing positions in an experimental work landscape.

Whether these new ideas will catch on is unknown. If lightweight portable electronic devices seamlessly linked to an internet of things provide us with all that we need to carry out our tasks then the need for chairs and desks, or rather the *affordances* provided by chairs and desks may become redundant, in which case all that may be needed are places for people to meet when they need to. The furniture and fittings most appropriate for the workspaces of the future will depend on the nature of the work to be done and tools available to do it. At the time of writing, these are unknown, but the affordance workspace may give us some clues.

What we do know though, is that our current state of knowledge is such that whatever work in the offices of the future looks like, we know enough to make it healthier than the offices of today by providing the *affordances* for natural postures and movements as seen in everyday life.

As Kevin Kelly of *Wired Magazine* has said:

> *The problem of the future will not be that we cannot connect – it will be that we cannot disconnect.*

# References

Adams, M.A., Bogduk, N., Burton, K. and Dolan, P. 2002. *The Biomechanics of Back Pain*. Churchill-Livingstone, Edinburgh.

Agarwal, S., Steinmaus, C. and Harris-Adamson, C. 2018. Sit-stand workstations and impact on low back discomfort: A systematic review and meta-analysis. *Ergonomics*, *61*(4), pp. 538–552.

Akerblom, B.A. 1954. Chairs and sitting: Symposium on human factors in equipment design. In Floyd, W.F. and Welford, A.T. (eds), *The Ergonomics Research Society, Proceedings, Vol II* (pp. 29–35). H.K. Lewis, London.

Alberti, K.G.M.M., Zimmet, P. and Shaw, J. 2006. Metabolic syndrome: A new world-wide definition. A consensus statement from the international diabetes federation. *Diabetic Medicine*, *23*(5), pp.469–480.

Arksey, H. 1988. *RSI and the Experts: The Construction of Medical Knowledge*. CRC Press, Boco Raton, Florida.

Banich, M.T. 2009. Executive function: The search for an integrated account. *Current Directions in Psychological Science*, *18*(2), pp. 89–94.

Basmajian, J.V. 1978. *Muscles Alive: Their Functions Revealed by Electromyography*, 4th edn. Williams and Wilkins, Baltimore.

Baumeister, R.F., Bratslavsky, E., Muraven, M. and Tice, D.M. 1998. Ego depletion: Is the active self a limited resource? *Journal of Personality and Social Psychology*, *74*(5), pp. 1252–1265.

Baumeister, R.F., Vohs, K.D. and Tice, D.M. 2007. The strength model of self-control. *Current Directions in Psychological Science*, *16*(6), pp. 351–355.

Belczak, C.E.Q., Belczak, S.Q., de Godoy, J.M.F., Ramos, R.N., de Oliveira, M.A. and Caffaro, R. A. 2009. Rate of occupational leg swelling is greater in the morning than in the afternoon. *Phlebology* (24), pp. 21–25.

Bendix, T. and Bridger, R.S. 2004. Seating Concepts. In Delleman, N., Haslegrave, C. and Chaffin, D. (eds), *Working Postures and Movements*. CRC Press: Fl, USA.

Bergouignan, A., Rudwill, F., Simon, C. and Blanc, S. 2011. Physical inactivity as the culprit of metabolic inflexibility: evidence from bed-rest studies. *Journal of applied physiology*, *111*(4), pp. 1201–1210.

Berman, M.G., Jonides, J. and Kaplan, S. 2008. The cognitive benefits of interacting with nature. *Psychological Science*, *19*(12), pp. 1207–1212.

Betts, J.A., Smith, H.A., Johnson-Bonson, D.A., Ellis, T.I., Dagnall, J., Hengist, A., Carroll, H., Thompson, D., Gonzalez, J.T. and Afman, G.H. 2018. The energy cost of sitting versus standing naturally in man. *Medicine and Science in Sports and Exercise*, April *51*(4), pp. 726–733.

Blumberg, B.S. amd Sokoloff, L. 1961. Coalescence of caudal vertebrae in the giant dinosaur diplodocus. *Arthritis and Rheumatism*, 4, pp. 592–601.

Bradbury, A., Evans, C., Allan, P., Lee, A., Ruckley, C.V. and Fowkes, F.G.R. 1999. What are the symptoms of varicose veins? Edinburgh vein study cross sectional population survey. *British Medical Journal*, *318*(7180), pp. 353–356.

Bridger, R.S. 2018. *Introduction to Human Factors and Ergonomics*, 4th edn. CRC Press, Boca Raton, Fl.

Bridger, R.S. and Orkin, D. 1992. Effect of a footrest on pelvic angle in stance. *Ergonomics SA*, pp. 42–48.

Bridger, R.S., Bennett, A. and Brasher, K. 2011. *Lifestyle, Body Mass Index and Self-Reported Health in the Royal Navy 2007–2011*. Unpublished MOD report.

Bridger, R.S., Brasher, K. and Bennett, A. 2013. Sustaining person-environment fit with a changing workforce. *Ergonomics, special issue on Ergonomics and Sustainability, 55*, pp. 565–577.

Bridger, R.S., Kloote, C., Rowlands, B. and Fourie, G. 2000. Palliative interventions for sedentary low back pain: The kneeling chair, the physiotherapy ball and conventional ergonomics compared. *Proceedings of HFES/IEA 2000* organized by the Human Factors and Ergonomics Society.

Bridger, R.S., Orkin, D. and Henneberg, M. 1992a. A quantitative investigation of lumbar and pelvic postures in standing and sitting: interrelationships with body position and hip muscle length. *International Journal of Industrial Ergonomics. 9*, pp. 235–244.

Bridger, R.S., Orkin, D., Henneberg, M. and Schierhout, G. 1992b. Investigations of posture in first and third world settings. The Ergonomics Society Conference, University of Aston, Birmingham, UK, April, 7–10.

Bridger, R.S., Verweccken, B., Whistance, R.S. and Adams, L.P. 1994. A prototype standing workspace. University of Warwick, Coventry, UK. In Robertson, S.A. (ed.), *Proceedings – Contemporary Ergonomics '94*, (pp. 482–487), Taylor and Francis, London.

Brownell, K. 2011. Is there courage to change America's diet? *Observer, 24*, pp. 15–17, Association for Psychological Science.

Buckley, J.P., Mellor, D.D., Morris, M. and Joseph, F. 2014. Standing-based office work shows encouraging signs of attenuating postprandial glycemic excursion. *Occupational and Environmental Medicine, 71*(2), pp. 109–111.

Burgerstein, L. and Netolitzky, A. 1985. *Handbuch der Schulhygiene*. Jena, Verlag Von Gustav Fischer.

Center for Disease Control. 2017. Long-term Trends in Diabetes April 2017. CDC's Division of Diabetes Translation. United States Diabetes Surveillance System, available at www.cdc.gov/diabetes/data

Cheema, J., Triglav, J., Strzalkowski, N., Howe, E. and Bent, L. 2017. *Physiological and Cognitive Measures During Prolonged Sitting: Comparisons Between a Standard and Multi-Axial Office Chair. A Preliminary Report*. University of Guleph.

Commissaris, D.A.C.M., Konemann, R., Hiemstra-van Mastrigt, S., Burford, E-M., Botter, J., Douwes, M. and Ellegast, R. 2014. Effects of a standing and three dynamic workstations on computer task performance and cognitive function tests. *Applied Ergonomics, 45*, pp. 1570–1578.

Commissaris, D.A.C.M., Huysmans, M.A., Mathiassen, S.E., Srinivasan, D., Koppes, L.L.J. and Hendriksen, I.J.M. 2016. Interventions to reduce sedentary behavior and increase physical activity during productive work: A systematic review. *Scandinavian Journal of Work, Environment & Health, 42*(3), pp. 181–191.

Cox, R., Shephard, J. and Corey, P. 1981. Influence of an employee fitness programme upon fitness, productivity and absenteeism. *Ergonomics, 24*, pp. 795–806.

Crum, A.J. and Langer, E.J. 2007. Mind-set matters: Exercise and the placebo effect. *Psychological Science, 18*, pp. 165–171.

Delleman, N.J. and Dul, J. 2007. International standards on working postures and movements ISO 11226 and EN 1005–4. *Ergonomics, 50*(11), pp. 1809–1819.

Dempster, W.T. 1955. The anthropometry of body action. *Annals of the New York Academy of Sciences*, pp. 559–585.

Dietrich, A. and Sparling, P.B. 2004. Endurance exercise selectively impairs prefrontal-dependent cognition. *Brain and Cognition, 55*(3), pp. 516–524.

Dul, J., Douwes, M. and Miedema, M. 1993. A guideline for the prevention of discomfort in static postures. In Nielsen, R. and Jorgensen, K. (eds), *Advances in Industrial Ergonomics and Safety*, (pp. 419–429), Taylor and Francis, London.

Dunstan, D.W., Kingwell, B.A., Larsen, R., Healy, G.N., Cerin, E., Hamilton, M.T., Shaw, J.E., Bertovic, D.A., Zimmet, P.Z., Salmon, J. and Owen, N. 2012. Breaking up prolonged sitting reduces postprandial glucose and insulin responses. *Diabetes Care*, p.DC_111931.

Dupont, F., Léger, P.M., Begon, M., Lecot, F., Sénécal, S., Labonté-Lemoyne, E. and Mathieu, M.E. 2019. Health and productivity at work: which active workstation for which benefits: a systematic review. *Occupational and Environmental Medicine*, *0*, pp. 1–14. DOI:10.1136/oemed-2018-105397

Fahrni, W.H. 1966. *Backache Relieved Through New Concepts in Posture*. Charles C. Thomas, Springfield, Il.

Fahrni, W.H. and Trueman, G. 1965. Comparative radiological study of the spines of a primitive population with North Americans, northern Europeans. *Journal of Bone and Joint Surgery*, *47B*, pp. 552–555.

Foster, R.S., Adams, L.P., van Geems, B. and Bridger, R.R. 1998. Postural adaptations to standing VDT work. *Occupational Ergonomics*, *1*(2), pp. 145–156.

Gailliot, M.T. 2015. Energy and Psychology. *Global Journal for Research Analytics*, *4*, pp. 253–255.

Gao, S., Zhai, Y., Yang, L., Zhang, H. and Gao, Y. 2018. Preferred temperature with standing and treadmill workstations. *Building and Environment*, *138*, pp. 63–73.

Garrett, G., Benden, M., Mehta, R., Pickens, A., Peres, S.C. and Zhao, H. 2016. Call center productivity over 6 months following a standing desk intervention. *IIE Transactions on Occupational Ergonomics and Human Factors*, *4*(2–3), pp. 188–195.

Garrett. G., Zhao, H., Pickens, A., Ranjana, M., Preston, L., Powell, A., Benden, M. 2019. Computer-based Prompt's impact on postural variability and sit-stand desk usage behavior; a cluster randomized control trial. *Applied Ergonomics*, *79*, pp. 17–24.

Gibson, J.J. 1979. *The Ecological Approach to Visual Perception*. Houghton Mifflin Harcourt (HMH), Boston.

Goetzel, R., Sepulveda, M., Knight, K., Eisen, M., Wade, S., Wong, J. and Fielding, J. 1994. Association of IBM's "A Plan for Life" health promotion programme with changes in employees' health risk status. *Journal of Occupational Medicine*, *36*, pp. 1005–1009.

Grandjean, E. 1973. *Ergonomics of the Home*. Taylor and Francis, London.

Grandjean, E. 1980. *Fitting the Task to the Man: A Textbook of Occupational Ergonomics*. Taylor and Francis, London.

Greer, A.E., Sui, X., Maslow, A.L., Greer, B.K. and Blair, S.N. 2015. The effects of sedentary behavior on metabolic syndrome independent of physical activity and cardiorespiratory fitness. *Journal of Physical Activity and Health*, *12*(1), pp. 68–73.

Gregory, D.E., Dunk, N.M. and Callaghan, J.P. 2006. Stability ball versus office chair: Comparison of muscle activation and lumbar spine posture during prolonged sitting. *Human Factors*, *48*(1), pp. 142–153.

Hales, C.M., Fryar, C.D., Carroll, M.D., Freedman, D.S. and Ogden, C.L. 2018. Trends in obesity and severe obesity prevalence in US youth and adults by sex and age, 2007–2008 to 2015–2016. *Jama*, *319*(16), pp. 1723–1725, DOI: 10.1001/jama.2018.3060.

Hardman, A.E., Hudson, A., Jones, P.R.M. and Norgan, N.G. 1989. Brisk walking and plasma cholesterol concentration in previously sedentary women. *British Medical Journal*, *299*, pp. 1204–1205.

Hart, G., 1998, September. Stand on sitting. What science has to say about seating options. In Global ergonomics. Proceedings of the Ergonomics Conference, South Africa. Cape Town: Elsevier (pp. 361–6).

Hartvigsen, J., Lebouef-Yde, C., Lings, S. and Corder, E. 2000. Is sitting-while-at-work associated with low back pain: A systematic, critical review of the literature. *Scandinavian Journal of Public Health*, *28*, pp. 231–239.

Healy, G.N., Dunstan, D.W., Salmon, J., Cerin, E., Shaw, J.E., Zimmet, P.Z. and Owen, N., 2008. Breaks in sedentary time: Beneficial associations with metabolic risk. *Diabetes Care*, *31*(4), pp.661–666.

Hellebrandt, F.A. 1938. Standing as a geotropic reflex. *American Journal of Physiology*, 121, pp. 471–474.

Hellebrandt, F.A. and Franseen, E.B. 1943. Physiological study of the vertical stance of man. *Physiological Reviews*, *23*(3), pp. 220–255.

Hewes, G.W. 1957. The anthropology of posture. *Scientific American*, *196*, pp. 122–132.

Hinton, D.C., Cheng, Y.Y. and Paquette, C. 2018. Everyday multitasking habits: University students seamlessly text and walk on a split-belt treadmill. *Gait & Posture*, *59*, pp. 168–173.

Hutchinson, A.D. and Wilson, C. 2012. Improving nutrition and physical activity in the workplace: A meta-analysis of intervention studies. *Health Promotion International*, *27*(2), pp. 238–249.

Kalichman, L. and Hunter, D.J. 2008. The genetics of intervertebral disc degeneration. Familial predisposition and heritability estimation. *Joint, Bone, Spine*, *75*(4), pp. 383–387.

Kaplan, S. 1995. The restorative benefits of nature: Toward an integrative framework. *Journal of Environmental Psychology*, *15*(3), pp. 169–182.

Karakolis, T., Barrett, J. and Callaghan, J.P. 2016. A comparison of trunk biomechanics, musculoskeletal discomfort and productivity during simulated sit-stand office work. *Ergonomics*, *59*(10), pp. 1275–1287.

Katzmarzyk, P.T., Church, T.S., Craig, C.L. and Bouchard, C., 2009. Sitting time and mortality from all causes, cardiovascular disease, and cancer. *Medicine & Science in Sports & Exercise*, *41*(5), pp. 998–1005.

Keegan, J.J. 1953. Alterations of the lumbar curve related to posture and seating. *Journal of Bone and Joint Surgery*, 35A, pp. 589–603.

Knight, K.K., Goetzel, R.Z., Fielding, J.E., Esien, M., Jackson, G.W., Kahr, T.Y., Kenny, G.M., Wade, S.W. and Duann, S. 1994. An evaluation of Duke University's LIVE FOR LIFE health program on changes in worker absenteeism. *Journal of Occupational Medicine*, *36*, pp. 533–536.

Koepp, G.A., Moore, G.K. and Levine, J.A. 2016. Chair-based fidgeting and energy expenditure. *British Medical Journal Open Sport & Exercise Medicine*, *2*(1), p.e000152.

Konz, S. and Johnson, S. 2007. *Work Design: Occupational Ergonomics.* CRC Press, Boca Raton, Fl.

Krijnen, R.M., de Boer, E.M., Adèr, H.J., Osinga, D.S. and Bruynzeel, D.P. 1997. Compression stockings and rubber floor mats: do they benefit workers with chronic venous insufficiency and a standing profession? *Journal of Occupational and Environmental Medicine*, *39*(9), pp. 889–894.

Lee, C.M., Jeong, E.H. and Freivalds, A. 2001. Biomechanical effects of wearing high-heeled shoes. *International Journal of Industrial Ergonomics*, *28*(6), pp. 321–326.

Lovejoy, C.O. 1988. Evolution of human walking. *Scientific American*, *259*, pp.118–125.

Luger, T., Cobb, T.J., Seibt, R., Rieger, M.A. and Steinhilber, B. 2019. Subjective evaluation of a passive lower-limb industrial exoskeleton used during simulated assembly. *IISE Transactions on Occupational Ergonomics and Human Factors*, (recently accepted), pp. 1–13.

Magora, A. 1972. Investigation of the relationship between low back pain and occupation. *Industrial Medicine*, *39*, pp. 504–510.

Mandal, A.C. 1987. *"The Seated Man" (homo sedens)*. Dafnia Publications, Taarbæk Strandvej 49, Klampenborg, Denmark.

Manohar, C., Levine, J.A., Nandy, D.K., Saad, A., Dalla Man, C., McCrady-Spitzer, S.K., Basu, R., Cobelli, C., Carter, R.E., Basu, A. and Kudva, Y.C. 2012. The effect of walking on postprandial glycemic excursion in patients with type 1 diabetes and healthy people. *Diabetes Care*, *35*(12), pp. 2493–2499.

Mansoubi, M., Pearson, N., Clemes, S.A., Biddle, S.J., Bodicoat, D.H., Tolfrey, K., Edwardson, C.L. and Yates, T. 2015. Energy expenditure during common sitting and standing tasks: Examining the 1.5 MET definition of sedentary behaviour. *BMC Public Health, 15*(1), p. 516.

McEwan, B.T., McDonald, D.J. and Burr, J.F. 2015. A systematic review of standing and treadmill desks in the workplace. *Preventative Medicine, 70*, pp. 50–58.

McGill, S.M., Kavcic, N.S. and Harvey, E. 2006. Sitting on a chair or an exercise ball: various perspectives to guide decision making. *Clinical Biomechanics, 21*(4), pp. 353–360.

Melzack, R. 1977. *The Puzzle of Pain.* Penguin Books Ltd., Harmondsworth, Middlesex, England.

Milne, R.A. and Mireau, D.R. 1979. Hamstring distensibility in the general population. Relationship to pelvic and low-back stress. *Journal of Manipulative and Physiological Therapeutics, 2*, pp. 146–150.

Nachemson, A. 1966. The load on the lumbar discs in different positions of the body. *Clinical Orthopaedics, 45*, pp. 107–122.

Nenonen, S., Rahtola, R. and Kojo, I. 2016. Third places and user preferences: Affordances in the cities. *Proceedings of CFM's Second Nordic Conference: Facilities Management Research and Practice*, August 29–30, 2016, Denmark. Jensen, P.A. (toim.).

Paffenbarger, R.S., Hyde, R.T., Jung, D.I. and Wing, A.I. 1984. Epidemiology of exercise and coronary heart disease. *Clinics in Sports Medicine, 3*, pp. 297–318.

Parikh, N.I., Pencina, M.J., Wang, T.J., Lanier, K.J., Fox, C.S., D'Agostino, R.B. and Vasan, R.S. 2007. Increasing trends in incidence of overweight and obesity over 5 decades. *The American Journal of Medicine, 120*(3), pp. 242–250.

Parry, S., Straker, L., Gilson, N.D. and Smith, A.J. 2013. Participatory workplace interventions can reduce sedentary time for office workers: A randomised controlled trial. *PloS one, 8*(11), p.e78957.

Paul, R.D. 1995. Foot swelling in VDT operators with sitting and sit-stand workstations. In *Proceedings of the Human Factors and Ergonomics Society Annual Meeting,* Vol. 39, October (10), pp. 568–572. Sage Publications, Los Angeles, CA.

Peddie, M.C., Bone, J.L., Rehrer, N.J., Skeaff, C.M., Gray, A.R. and Perry, T.L. 2013. Breaking prolonged sitting reduces postprandial glycemia in healthy, normal-weight adults: A randomized crossover trial. *American Journal of Clinical Nutrition, 98*(2), pp.358–366.

Proença, M., Schuna Jr, J.M., Barreira, T.V., Hsia, D.S., Pitta, F., Tudor-Locke, C., Cowley, A.D. and Martin, C.K. 2018. Worker acceptability of the Pennington Pedal Desk™ occupational workstation alternative. *Work*, (Preprint), pp. 1–8.

Robert Wood Johnson Foundation. 2018. The State of Obesity: Physical inactivity in the United States, available at https://www.stateofobesity.org/physical-inactivity/

Robertson, M.M., Ciriello, V.R. and Garabet, A.M. 2012. Office ergonomics training and a sit-stand workstation: Effects on musculoskeletal and visual symptoms and performance of office workers. *Applied Ergonomics, 44*(2013), pp. 73–85.

Rogers, Y. and Rodden, T. 2002. Designing new workspaces to provide physical and social affordances for successful interaction. In Workshop paper presented at CSCW, available at http://citeseerx.ist.psu.edu/viewdoc/download?doi=10.1.1.591.3906&rep=rep1&type=pdf.

Rynders, C.A., Blanc, S., DeJong, N., Bessesen, D.H. and Bergouignan, A. 2018. Sedentary behaviour is a key determinant of metabolic inflexibility. *Journal of Physiology, 596*(8), pp. 1319–1330.

Rys, M. and Konz, S. 1989. An evaluation of floor surfaces. In *Proceedings of the Human Factors Society Annual Meeting*, Vol. 33, October (8), pp. 517–520. Sage Publications: Los Angeles, CA.

Rys, M. and Konz, S. 1994. Standing. *Ergonomics, 37*(4), pp. 677–687.

Satzler, L., Satzler, C. and Konz, S. 1993. Standing aids. Proceedings of the Ayoub Sympoium, Texas Tech University, Lubboch, TX 29–31.

Scholey, A., Macpherson, H., Sünram-Lea, S., Elliott, J., Stough, C. and Kennedy, D. 2013. Glucose enhancement of recognition memory: Differential effects on effortful processing but not aspects of "remember-know" responses. *Neuropharmacology, 64*, pp. 544–549.

Schuna, J.M., Hsia, D.S., Tudor-Locke, C., Johannsen, N.M. 2019. Energy expenditure while using workstation alternatives at self-selected intensities. *Journal of Physical Activity and Health, 16*(2), pp. 141–148.

Semmer N., Zapf D. and Dunckel H. 1995. Assessing stress at work: A framework and an instrument. In Svane, C. and Johansen, O. (ed.), *Work and Health: Scientific Basis of Progress* in *the Working Environment*, (pp. 105–113) Office for Official Publications of the European Communities; Luxembourg.

Sen, R.N. 1984. Application of ergonomics in industrially developing countries. The Ergonomics Society, The Society's Lecture, 1983, reprinted in *Ergonomics, 27*(10), pp. 1021–1032.

Shaw, A.M., Wootton, S.A., Fallowfield, J.L., Allsopp, A.J. and Parsons, E.L. 2019. Environmental interventions to promote healthier eating and physical activity behaviours in institutions: a systematic review. *Public Health Nutrition*, pp. 1–14.

Sherrington, C.S. 1933. *The Brain and its Mechanism*. Cambridge University Press.

Shorland, F.B. 1988. Is our knowledge of human nutrition soundly based? *World Reviews of Nutrition and Dietetics, 57*, pp. 126–205.

Shrestha, N., Ijaz, S., Kukkonen-Harjula, K.T., Kumar, S. and Nwankwo, C.P. 2015. *Workplace Interventions for Reducing Sitting at Work (Review)*. The Cochrane Collaboration published by John Wiley and Sons Ltd.

Sluiter, J.K., de Croon, E.M., Meijman, T. and Frings-Dresen, M. 2003. Need for recovery from work-related fatigue and its role in the development and prediction of subjective health complaints. *Occupational and Environmental Medicine, 60*(Suppl I, i-62–i70).

Smith, J.W. 1953. The act of standing, *Acta Orthopaedica Scandinavica, 23*, pp. 159–168.

Smith, L., Sawyer, A., Gardner, B., Seppala, K., Ucci, M., Marmot, A., Lally, P. and Fisher, A. 2018. Occupational physical activity habits of UK office workers: Cross-sectional data from the active buildings study. *International Journal of Environmental Research and Public Health, 15*(6), p. 1214.

Snijders, C.J., Slagter, A.H., Vleeming, A., Stoeckart, R. and Stam, H.J. 1995. Why leg crossing? The influence of common postures on abdominal muscle activity. *Spine, 20*(18), pp. 1989–1993.

Son, J.I., Yi, C.H., Kwon, O.Y., Cynn, H.S., Lim, O.B., Baek, Y.J. and Jung, Y.J. 2018. Effects of footrest heights on muscle fatigue, kinematics, and kinetics during prolonged standing work. *Journal of Back and Musculoskeletal Rehabilitation*, (Preprint), pp. 1–8.

Speksnijder, C.M., vd Munckhof, R.J., Moonen, S.A. and Walenkamp, G.H. 2005. The higher the heel the higher the forefoot-pressure in ten healthy women. *The Foot, 15*(1), pp. 17–21.

Staffcl, F. 1884. Zur Hygieine des Sitzens (The hygiene of sitting). *Zefltr AI/gem Gest/ ndheitspflege, 3*, pp. 403–421.

Straker, L. and Mathiassen, M. 2009. Increased physical work loads in modern work: A necessity for better health and performance. *Ergonomics, 52*, pp. 1215–1225.

Strasser, H. 1913. Lehrbuch der Muskel- und Gelenkmechanik, 2. In Akerblom, B. (ed.) *Standing and Sitting Posture*. Thesis: Stockholm, 1948.

Sundstrom, E. 1986. *Workplaces*. Cambridge University Press.

Taylor, F.W. 1911. *The Principles of Scientific Management*. Harper and Brothers Publishers, New York and London.

Thompson, W.O., Thompson, P.K. and Dailey, M.E. 1928. The effect of posture upon the composition and volume of the blood in man. *Journal of Clinical Investigation, 5*(4), pp. 573–604.

Tomei, F., Baccolo, T.P., Palmi, S. and Rosati, M.V. 1999. Chronic venous disorders and occupation. *American Journal of Industrial Medicine, 36*, pp. 653–665.

Tuchsen, F., Krause, N., Hannerz, H. and Burr, T.S. 2000. Standing at work and varicose veins. *Scandinavian Journal of Work, Environment & Health, 26*(5), pp. 414–420.

Van der Ploeg, H.P., Chey, T., Korda, R.J., Banks, E. and Bauman, A. 2012. Sitting time and all-cause mortality risk in 222 497 Australian adults. *Archives of Internal Medicine*, *172*(6), pp. 494–500.

Venema, T.A., Kroese, F.M. and De Ridder, D.T. 2018. I'm still standing: A longitudinal study on the effect of a default nudge. *Psychology & Health*, *33*(5), pp. 669–681.

Vink, P., Konijn, I., Jongejan, B. and Berger, M. 2009. Varying the office work posture between standing, half-standing and sitting results in less discomfort. In *International Conference on Ergonomics and Health Aspects of Work with Computers* July. (pp. 115–120). Springer, Berlin, Heidelberg.

Wen, C.P., Wai, J.P.M., Tsai, M.K., Yang, Y.C., Cheng, T.Y.D., Lee, M.C., Chan, H.T., Tsao, C.K., Tsai, S.P. and Wu, X. 2011. Minimum amount of physical activity for reduced mortality and extended life expectancy: a prospective cohort study. *The Lancet*, *378*(9798), pp. 1244–1253.

Wilmot, E.G., Edwardson, C.L., Achana, F.A., Davies, M.J., Gorely, T., Gray, L.J., Khunti, K., Yates, T. and Biddle, S.J. 2012. Sedentary time in adults and the association with diabetes, cardiovascular disease and death: systematic review and meta-analysis. *Diabetologia*, *55*(1), pp. 2895–2905.

Whistance, R.S., Adams, L.P., Geems, B.V. and Bridger, R.S. 1995. Postural adaptations to workbench modifications in standing workers. *Ergonomics*, *38*(12), pp. 2485–2503.

White, A.A. and Panjabi, M.M. 1990. *Clinical Biomechanics of the Spine* (Vol. 2, pp. 108–112). Lippincott, Philadelphia.

Wrege, C.D. and Greenwood, R.G. 1991. *Frederick W. Taylor, the Father of Scientific Management: Myth and Reality*. Irwin Professional Pub., Homewood, Il.

Ying Gao, Nevala, N., Cronin, N.J., Finni, T. 2016. Effects of environmental intervention on sedentary time, musculoskeletal comfort and work ability in office work. *European Journal of Sports Science*, *16*(6), pp. 747–754.

Zacharow, D. 1988. *Posture: Sitting, Standing, Chair Design and Exercise*. Charles C. Thomas, Springfield, Il.

# Index

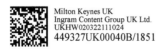